To
Karen

I pray
for you always.

[signature] 5/1/04

Back From The Edge

By

Jorge Joseph Taylor

authorHOUSE

1663 Liberty Drive, Suite 200
Bloomington, Indiana 47403
(800) 839-8640
www.authorhouse.com

First published by AuthorHouse 07/15/04

ISBN: 1-4184-0761-5 (e)
ISBN: 1-4184-0760-7 (sc)

Printed in the United States of America
Bloomington, Indiana

This book is printed on acid-free paper.

Edited by: Michel V. Wheeler.

Sometimes I Struggle

By Soledad Taylor Churchill

Sometimes it's hard; I struggle
Just to see the light of day
To feel the sun against my skin,

Just to feel the comfort of another
To feel like I belong somewhere,

Sometimes I struggle; it's all I know
I feel like I need to get away

But not to hide
Just some space and or little time,

Until I can bring myself to look within
Just to peek at what's inside

Dedication

I dedicate this book to my beautiful wife, The Reverend Jennie L. Taylor, for her love and support throughout the course of my illness. Words are not enough to express the measure of love that flows from my heart for her. I love her with all the love in my heart.

I dedicate this book to my children. They are the flowers in the garden of my life.

I thank God for granting me stewardship over my daughter Tina, her husband Chris and their son Isaac, my daughter Camille, her husband Tracy and their twin girls, Treasure and Tasia, and her sons Micah and Tahjj. I thank God for my son, Jorge II, his wife Debra and his daughter Jacqueline, and his son, Mikael. I thank God for my sons Miguel, Armando, his girl friend Corrie and the newest flower in the Taylor garden, baby Ashlee.

I dedicate this book to all my brothers and sisters that must persevere in the midst of the circumstances in the world of dialysis, and all of you with similar fate and challenges to be overcome in your lives.

Acknowledgment

I have promised just about every member of my family that I would give an account of my trip to the edge. They seem to be convinced that somewhere in this experience there is a story worth revealing. I suppose they could be right, but I must warn you that these accounts aren't really my own. I am merely the messenger. You see, I was either at the edge of my consciousness, or on my way back from it when these occurrences took place.

The information recorded here in "Back from the Edge" was made possible because of the contribution of the numerous dialysis patients, and professionals I encountered on this journey.

I am indebted to Dr. Geofrey Block, a man of compassion and dedication to his patients and to his profession. Dr. Block is not only my nephrologists, but he is the chief medical officer at the Lowry Dialysis Center, a member of the Davita community in Denver. I must also recognize its Former Facility Administrator, Gary E. Hamilton.

A special thanks to The Gambro Dialysis Care Center in Henderson, North Carolina, and the National Kidney Foundation for its statistical information.

Had it not been for the prayers and support of my co-workers at Avaya Communications, and a host of friends that kept me lifted up before the Lord; had it not been for the support of my Mt. Gilead Baptist Church family, and its staff: Bishop Acen Phillips, my Pastor Rev. Del T. Phillips, and Dr. Walter Hill Jr., my family, and friends here in Colorado and across the nation, I would not be able to promote these pages of testimony.

I take this opportunity to thank all of you from the bottom of my heart, and I pray for God's continued blessing on all your lives.

I want to acknowledge the following members of my family and dearest friends whose support played a major role in my coping strategy; my sisters, Anita, Taylor and, Debbie, my mother Hazel Headley, my brother John and his wife Patsy, my Uncle George and his wife Sylvia, my cousins Celina, Cecilia, and Miguel, my wife's mother Millie Alston, and in the living memory of her deceased father, Floyd Alston. I acknowledge my friends Calvin and Sandra Lucky, James and Michele Wheeler, Burvell and Susie Williams, Fred and Pearl Jones, my prayer warrior Sheila Barnes, and in memory of the late Deacon Charles Massey.

In conclusion, it is my prayer that the salvation of our Lord Jesus Christ comes to all. Let it further be known that should anyone read the words in this book and find consolation, strength, encouragement, or inspiration to sustain them in their faith and their circumstances, then, let the glory of this testimony be to Our Lord and Savior Jesus Christ.

Introduction

Because I was unable to prevent the experiences that lead to my demise, some would want to label me a victim of circumstances, but you are probably familiar with the expression, "God takes care of fools and babies". Well, I'm here to add that he also takes care of grown ups who find themselves surrendered to slumber through it all.

My experiences at the edge are expressed in two distinct and separate sequences of events. The first sequence depicts the period of discovery of ESRD End (Stage Renal Disease), hypertension, a collapsed lung, and a mass found on my left kidney.

During a two week hospitalization period, I was diagnosed as having all of the above ailments. Not as apparent though was the encroachment or disturbance to my spirit, my emotions, my subconscious, my dream world.

The second sequence of this book depicts surviving and coping with (ESRD). This is the post hospitalization period of my illness. It is where treatment begins. For some dialysis patients, this period can last anywhere from a year to twenty years or, for many, it can be a lifetime experience.

The entries for this sequence of events are expressed in memoir or diary form. I must explain that at the time of this publication there is no known cure for the loss of a kidney. The best that one can do is to continue the services that the kidney once provided the body with the use of a dialysis machine. I must also inform you that without these services the body would be poisoned by the by-product of its own toxic wastes and eventually die.

Becoming aware of the loss of a kidney can be an emotionally confusing time. It seems like a chunk of time has been extracted from one's life with no explanation whatsoever. The expression, "You never miss the water until the well runs dry", is ever so true. Not only do you never miss the water, better yet, you never even knew that the well itself ever existed. It is like becoming an adult and realizing that even though the acquisition of food and shelter never concerned us as children, they were never an option. It feels as if the innocence of childhood has been violated, stolen, and now we must be forever vigilant as we learn how to counter the agenda and strategies of this disease. Those of us who have experienced this circumstance must learn to co-exist inside our bodies with a thief who comes to steal our body parts and destroy our lives.

Accepting our circumstances is critical to the successful development of a coping strategy. Keep in mind that this does not mean surrendering or giving up the fight.

On the contrary, it means that we must assess our position, learn the do's and don'ts, and dig in for the stand of our life. This is a time when we must demand endurance of our courage from minutes, to hours, and from days to months and even years if necessary. It is a time when the enemy invades our subconscious and establishes strongholds in our mind, putting our faith and beliefs to the test and stretching them like the rubber of a sling shot.

Having a support system of friends, family, the best healthcare professionals you can find, and last but not least, a team of relentless prayer warriors should be part of our arsenal. This is what I consider the coping essentials for a fighting chance against ESRD.

Table of Contents

Part I

1
Stroke Level

Jorge Joseph Taylor

One week before being admitted to the hospital, I went to see my family doctor with the most excruciating headache. He advised me that at 166 over 150 my blood pressure was a little too high, but nothing to be alarmed about. He then handed me a prescription for some painkillers and concluded our meeting with an appointment to return by the end of the month.

I really was not satisfied with the doctor's routine examination, because I knew that it was not going to cure my ailment. It was my duty to let him know how I felt, instead I just followed the doctor's orders as he suggested.

A few days later, I was forced into submission. I couldn't stand up against the pain any longer. It was the second episode of a debilitating headache that drove me first to my knees and then to assume a fetal position underneath my desk at work. I couldn't wait for an appointment at the end of the month. This was now ER (emergency room) time.

My son, Jorge II, drove the car the short distance to the hospital. After a long six year tour of duty, he had just returned home from the Marine Corp. We talked about many things and planned many projects that would move our lives to another level together. My oldest son and my oldest daughter are alike in this way. They are very graphic, very excitable and melodramatic. He was so very excited about being home. Wherever his life took him while

4

he was away, it was to become better now that he was home with his dad. He was excited about the things that we were going to set in motion together. He came home looking for the leadership and friendship of his father, and I disappointed him, instead he had to carry me. This was a psychological devastation to our relationship. Once upon a time he thought that coming home was the best course that his life could take. Now he talks about taking some work over seas in the rebuilding of Iraq. I am hopeful that some day we will be able to repair our feelings and then build a project together.

If you are not familiar with hospital admission procedure, or ER in particular, maybe you ought to try a dry run before having to go through the real thing. The time it took to get me registered and admitted was not very long, but that was only because my vital signs were reading off the charts. Had it not been for that fact, I assure you that I would have been waiting there for a couple of hours like the rest of unfortunates I saw.   Don't you think that because you are bleeding to death, you will be exempt from taking care of the two hours worth of admission dossier papers. Not so, you still must furnish two or three forms of ID, one must be a picture, current insurance card, and then you sign, and sign and sign in the fashion of a home closing. By the way, it is not such a bad Idea for you to memorize your mother's maiden name.

The nursing assistant flipped the blood pressure band around my arm in a most familiar and routine fashion. This nurse had done this procedure many times during her career with very similar results in the reading of the instrument. Not this time. This time would be different. This was that text-book case students read about, but maybe very few have the opportunity to actually experience it. I am sure that she was not aware that her jaw had dropped open, and her eyes remained fixed on the blood pressure instrument. She stopped, and looked around for someone to confirm what she had just read. No one else had seen those results but her. So she was forced to do it all over again. With her eyes fixed on the instrument, the nurse pumped the cup frantically, stopping only to release its pressure occasionally. Suddenly, she took off like a bat out of hell, and left me standing with the blood pressure cup dangling from my arm. Within seconds she was back. I was informed of the critical nature of my blood pressure reading 230/150. "Stroke level", she insisted. I was a stroke waiting to happen, and why I was still on my feet was a mystery to her. That was the last thing I remembered during the admission procedures.

When I look back on that day, it is hard to believe that the only thing that precipitated the life threatening events of the next two weeks was a splitting headache. One day I had a splitting headache, and that was the only real beginning of this experience, and no matter how hard

I try, I am unable to resolve or bring some closure to this experience not even in my mind. It reminds me of one of the dreams I had at the edge. Dreams with seemingly incomplete experiences; dreams that leaves you numb, bewildered, and longing for an end; a good example of this is the fifteen car pile up that I am about to describe.

2
Fifteen Car
Pile Up

Jorge Joseph Taylor

I knew that there was some sort of accident up ahead. Curiosity was getting the best of me. Traffic was at a stand still, and I just had to know what was backing it up like this. A fresh blanket of snow had just fallen over the city. Fluffy, glistening snow flakes rested undisturbed under the glow of the city's street lamps, but all the occupants remained inside the warmth and comfort of their automobiles. The rumbling sounds of idling engines dared to interrupt the peacefulness of the evening. That was the scenery; while we waited for the police to arrive.

If only I had enough room to maneuver my vehicle out of this line, not only would I be able to see what's holding us up but at the same time, I would be able to cut in the front of the line way up ahead. Well, that idea was out of the question, because our vehicles where packed in like harvested sardines. Not enough room to maneuver the car out of the line. My concentration on the wreckage up ahead was so focused that I actually willed my spirit up ahead of the traffic. This was so cool. I believe it is called teleportation; that is when your spirit levitates and leaves your body. What I saw when I got up to the head of the line was even crazier. The initial car had skidded into a vehicle and caused the chain reaction of a wreck involving some fifteen cars.

I approached the initial vehicle to see if anyone was hurt. I was shocked to find my physical self as a passenger along with a nurse who was preoccupied with reconnecting the electrodes wires that had become loose on my body. You know those electrode wires that they attach to your body in the telemetry ward for the purpose of reading ones vital signs! The nurse performed like a drone. I wanted to believe that her behavior was a result of this accident, but I can't really be sure.

Let me continue to relate the bizarre events. We are not quite finished yet. For some odd reason, I was becoming aware that this activity seemed to be unending. After focusing on these elements, I noticed that when the nurse finished hooking me back up to all the wires, one of her final acts was to administer to me some sort of medication, which put me out to pasture somewhere. I would somehow end up at the back of the line, which lead to a traffic jam that started this episode all over again. It wasn't a continuation, but rather a redundancy of events. Rather than appearing committed to her work, the nurse seemed more like a drone responding in a mechanical manner. I was imprisoned by these perpetual events, prolonged through the reappearance of an obedient nurse. A wake up call would not come any too soon. How else would I escape the plague of these unending events?

3
The E.R.
Experience

Dr. Ben Monroe, and Dr. Ron Knights, may God rest his soul; came to see me. It did my heart good to see them. We come from the same Alma Mater, The University of New Mexico. These two friends encouraged my spirit through my undergraduate years in college. Dr. Monroe said to me. "I bet you've got a new found respect for ER". He was referring to the television show, and of course, he was right. All I could do was to nod my head in response. It was very uncomfortable and difficult to swallow. It felt as if I had a two by four stuck down my throat. A breathing machine with the balloon was taped to my mouth, while some other contraption was placed inside of my chest to help keep my lungs inflated.

Thanks to the advent of television and the advancement of medicine, Joe Public has access to these procedures. In fact, it was a good thing that I had the memory from the TV show ER, because the experience that I paid for turned out to be a bit foggy with all the sedatives in my body.

My friend Ben, had no idea of how much on target he was. I do have a respect for the speed at which doctors make decisions, And yes, much of what I experienced in the hospital very closely resembled what I have seen on the television show ER. Or is it the other way around? I do owe my life to the sound judgment and quick reaction time of the professionals in the hospital.

Gratitude was the furthest thing from my mind while these people were performing their duty. As a matter of fact, you could not have convinced me that they were working in my behalf. I had the illusion that they were making me sicker. First of all I could not believe that I was as sick as they were saying I was. How could I, when all I had upon admission was a splitting headache, or so I thought.

After a couple days stay in the hospital, I noticed a host of flowers and get well cards left by friends seemed to all make reference to me giving them the scare of their life. Those were the exact words from my doctor's mouth as he walked around my bed burdened with the most exhausted look on his unshaven face. I had just gotten out of Intensive Care Unit, but everyone else carried my scars of extreme exhaustion.

It was not until later, much later, that I got the nerve to ask what did I do that scared them so. I knew that I was not your model patient. After all, I felt that these people were trying to keep me sedated, having me think that I was going crazy. I knew that I was sometimes rude to some of these people who were trying to help me. I really began to worry that I may have been offensive to someone. I just didn't have the nerves to ask what I had done. Actually, had I been told that I was less than a civilized person, and I had caused somebody some grief, I

Jorge Joseph Taylor

would not be able to deny it. I would have been forced to accept whatever I was told.

After being welcomed back to the regular ward, I was told by a nurse that she was so happy to see me back. My return back to a regular ward was nothing short of a miracle. People that spend as much time as I did in the Intensive Care Unit normally don't come back to the floor. What I mean is, they are hauled out in a pine box.

4
Out of Body Experience

I believe that I did leave my body for a moment, while in the intensive care unit. What caused my heart rate to take off like a Quarter Horse at the Belmont Stakes I don't know, and I don't believe that they, (the nurses and doctors taking care of me), knew either.

I could see the monitor and I could feel the thumping pressure in my body as the pace of my heartbeat escalated. The constant alarm of beeping noise made by all the vital machines embeds itself in your subconscious. Sometimes the attendants come to turn it off, but most times they just ignore them, and they just go on forever. That whole sterile environment smell of plastic tubes in your mouth, in your nose, in your throat, IV's stuck in your arm, hanging from your chest and all over your body, along with the smell of medications, saline and other intravenous fluids is an overwhelming experience to say the least.

A certain nurse looked at her partner questioningly, "What happened," she asked? They both jumped backwards away from my bed, as if they expected me to explode and were attempting to avoid getting hit by debris of body of body parts. It didn't take the duty nurse long to get a hold of herself and administer some medication through my IV.

My poor arm started to looked like a road map, just riddled with hypodermic needle pricks. I have been poked so much that my veins now roll and hide when a nurse or a technician shows up with a needle in hand. Almost

18

immediately, the medication took effect as my heart rate could be seen on the monitor subsiding.

I hovered above my bed. I could see the crowd of people that stood in prayer asking God to spare my life. I tried to get the attention of one of my coworkers. She looked directly at me, but somehow she could not see or hear me calling her. I tried to get her attention or anybody's for that matter to let them know that I was all right, that I wasn't dead. Communication between me and the world that I knew had been severely hampered. It was a strange moment. I had no knowledge of my body laying there, until I hovered high enough above the bed to be able to look down. All this time, I looked straight ahead at my coworkers who where praying and sobbing at the same time. I did not feel dead. Even when I called out at my friends, and they did not respond, it did not dawn on me that I might have been dead. Only after levitating high enough and moving towards the foot of the bed did I see myself and had the suspicion that something drastic had taken place.

It is to this day difficult to understand or place here or there. Maybe this crowd of people knew something that I could not see, because I really wasn't there. Maybe I was the only one in that room wondering outside of their body.

It took a while for me to understand that my wife had not placed me in the care of a private and exclusive facility.

Jorge Joseph Taylor

The medication that I was under had totally saturated my consciousness. I have memories of her staying with me at the mansion for several nights, and she was now going home to shower and get some rest. She reminded me that my mother was arriving that same night, and she would return after picking her up from the airport.

It seems like several hours had passed since she had left, and I started to get nervous. For a moment I thought I heard her voice out in the waiting room. After explaining my concern for my mother being picked up from the airport, I sent the nurse out to see if my wife had returned. The nurse came back after what seemed like a half hour with a smile on her face, she was ready to administer medication, but made no reference to my request. I became impatient and could not wait for her, so I asked about my wife. Her reply was, "What did you want? Oh, you want me to see if your wife is in the waiting area, right? I will check right away for you, sir." I realize that people do make mistakes and forget sometimes, and given the very mature age of this nurse I gave her the benefit of the doubt.

The second attempt to locate my wife was no different than the first, only this time, I went totally ballistic to the point of screaming at the top of my lungs, inviting other nurses and technicians to inquire about me. Well, needless to say, it wasn't long before a sedative was administered to me, and before I knew it, morning had come, and the daytime follows its own course of priorities.

During the daytime, my stay in the hospital followed a full schedule. Orderlies and nurses begin their morning at 4:30 a.m. as they wake you out of your nightmare to extract your blood. There are other nurses that administer medication through the night, and let's not forget the specialists such as the respiratory people. If you were like me, they were there every hour on the hour. No one was appointed to see that you got enough sleep or rest. Do not disturb signs do not exist in this environment. Let me qualify this statement. I don't want it to sound like this is all bad. There were times during my dreams when I would have given anything to have one of these night rider specialists, rescue me from the fate at the hands of the enforcer.

5
The
Enforcers

I was to meet the boys at the park for football practice. For some odd reason, our practice field was located near a down town business district. After arriving, I looked at my watch and noticed that I was a half hour late for football practice and not a single boy in sight. I began to search for the boys. Who knows what they may have gotten themselves in to. I had exhausted probably an hour in my search, and evening was running fast towards the horizon.

In this police state environment, it is not wise to be caught out in the street after dark. My wife and I managed to elude these fast moving Gestapo like troops. We crouched behind stair wells and hid in dark, treacherous alleys. We could hear the enforcer's boots pounding the pavement in unison during their double time patrol through the district. Military police trucks, delivery vehicles, mail trucks, and other commercial vehicles seem to dominate the traffic.

It was now dark and difficult to see. While attempting to stand up, I leaned against the wall. It gave away and I tumbled backwards through an opening, pulling my wife out of the alley. It was some sort of metal door. "Just as well", I thought.   I wasn't too crazy about the spot, but we had to settle down somewhere for the night to avoid being captured. The spot was very dark. We couldn't see our hands in front of us. It was very quiet you could hear a pin drop. We thought it might be best to keep it that way. We made our self as comfortable as possible and tried our best not to make a sound. Within minutes, I heard the voice of my daughter calling from somewhere out in the alley. I asked my wife if she heard it. She thought that she heard the sound of someone humming. On second thought, I did hear a sound of some sort of machine, but I can't be sure. I am concentrating on hearing my daughter's voice again and trying to figure out where it's coming from.

About the time that I heard the word "Dad" again, I felt a slight nudging pressure from the wall up against my back. "How can this be"? I thought. "Nothing is back there but the wall". With my fingers to my lips, I motioned to my wife to be quiet. It was that sound again. The one she thought was someone humming. At the same time the pressure against my back occurred again. "What the hell, something is back there", I whispered to my wife. There really wasn't anything there but the wall, and it was closing in on us.

We were sitting in the back of some sort of garbage compactor. I grabbed my wife by her arm and attempted to run. She resisted. I couldn't understand. She started to call for the nurse. I knew that would be trouble. The nurse usually gets there with her syringe drawn like a wild, wild, West character. My experiences with her seem to always end in defeat. I ended up getting stuck by her needle and drifting into la-la land.

Jorge Joseph Taylor

So, here I lay in this dumpster that is compacting and about to crush us alive. Should I manage to escape this trash compactor then I must confront the Borg Militia patrolling outside whose purpose is to assimilate everyone with the purpose of the collective. Of all the fate that awaited me: being crushed by the compactor, getting caught by the Militia, or facing the nurse somewhere at the edge of my consciousness, the latter, would be the most fearful of all.

I pleaded with my wife for dear life. "Please! Honey, please don't call the nurse! You know what will happen if the nurse comes over here. She will sedate me." I feared being sedated with a passion. I was put into an induced sleep and the dreams at the edge begin to play. The cycle of these dreams go on forever. Try as I may to wake up and get out of these dreams, some how I'm drawn right back to the beginning of the dreams.

6
Remembering
The Struggle

Jorge Joseph Taylor

Next to God, my family and friends are the most important aspects of my life. I don't know how I would have made it through this ordeal without them. My wife and all my children, except for my eldest daughter Tina, took turn staying with me overnight at the hospital. Tina was already there. She was two floors above me enduring a struggle of her own.

God is totally awesome. In the midst of my unexpected challenge, my daughter presented me with a brand spanking new grandchild, Isaac is his name. I am sure that you are aware that it is a biblical name meaning laughter. If for no other reason I must fight to experience the joy that this new birth will bring us.

I really had not realized until much later, what my family had been going through during this ordeal. My daughter, Camille explains it this way. "Dad, we were all boo hooing and praying with long solemn faces while we visited you. We would then run upstairs, within minutes of seeing you switching gears between the floors as we went, to see my sister and her beautiful new born baby. Can you imagine what it took to do that, Dad"?

My wife is not only a fighter; she is a teacher as well. She taught us how to persevere and survive the challenge. During her bout with cancer, I watched her resist the enemy. She persevered with radiation therapy treatment every other day for eight weeks. She just kept going until

28

the monster that attempted to grow inside her breast was subdued, and hopefully defeated.

Camille was not only like a breath of fresh air, but the ace up my sleeve of weapons in my recovery arsenal. She was the person that in my mind's eye held the key to my sanity and trust when everyone else seemed preoccupied with other issues. Please don't misunderstand what I am trying to say. I must be clear to you my reader.

I have been made to understand that some medication, especially the ones used for sedation, may have hallucinating effects on some people. Well, guess what, yours truly fits the model of some people perfectly. These medications, whatever their purpose, had me climbing the walls and hanging from the ceiling. They had taken over my mind. Certain individuals close to me, as in the case of my wife, became my enemies. Those in charge of the care of my health, became as wardens of an imprisonment facility.

I remember having just been sedated. The room that I was in was of glass. It reminded me of a Rubik's cube. I was having extreme difficulty distinguishing the ceiling and walls from the floor. I was able to walk up the sides of the walls. At times the walls would right themselves and become floors, and other times not. When this happened, I would find myself stuck to the walls and unable to get back to the floors. This was obviously a problem. Camille was visiting me during one of these episodes. She was

29

a God send to me. There were other people in the room visiting me. I just couldn't trust them not to involve the nurse. I leaned over to Camille and whispered in her ears asking her if she thought I was right side up, because I felt that I wasn't. I then told her to hold on to me so that I wouldn't transform.

The next incident that I confided in Camille was to tell her that I was about to go domestic. Not only was I going to cook my own food, henceforth, but I was going to be responsible for hunting my own meat as well. I hope that you are not expecting an explanation, because there isn't one. Camille did not ask for an explanation, except for how was I going to hunt my meat. I indicate that I was going to acquire the use of a bow and arrow. She acknowledged my comments by simply nodding her head. As I look back on the conversation we had, maybe they were not what you would call mainstream, but I am so glad that she was there to keep me sane.

My health took a critical turn for the worse when my lungs collapsed. I can remember standing and just getting very warm on the inside. The more difficult it was to breath, the warmer it seemed to get. It was as if the air that flowed through my lungs was also the system that regulated my body temperature. The shut down occurred rather quickly. The next thing I remember was not being able to hear any one speaking. I could see their lips moving but no sound. It was like watching a pantomime production. I could not hear a sound. I tried to convey my condition to my wife, who went to the nurse's station for help.

Signs of distress and panic were now overtaking my wife's expression. The nurse that returned kept telling me to take deep breaths. I kept trying to communicate that there was no air to get, and that I was suffocating. There was a slight struggle and finally things became blurry and unconsciousness prevailed.

I never knew what really happened that day until I ran into George. His peers regarded him as a nurse that was very much on top of his game. George passed by my room in a flash. Had it not been for his distinctive voice I would not have recognized the blur that went by my doorframe. He looked as if he had seen a ghost. He had a great big sunshine smile on his face that converted immediately into a frown.

"...And what are you still doing here"? He questioned me with great curiosity.   I explained to him that I had just been released from the Intensive Care Unit. "And you have been up there all this time?" I did not know all of what time he was referring to. As far as I was concerned, it all transpired within a day or two, but I answered ,"yes all this time." He knew that I had been up in Intensive Care, because he sent me there. He didn't expect that I would be there for almost a week.

"Well, you went through some complication, buddy. I want to ask you a question", George said, "This has been bugging me ever since you went up to ICU. "Tell me how much do you remember about what happened down here on the floor. What do you remember about me"? I didn't understand what he meant by his question. "How much had I remembered?"

"Do you remember the struggle you put up before you got sedated?" George looked at me with a questioning look on his face. "No" I answered. "It's a matter of fact there isn't much that I remember about that day." George looked at me with a smirk on his face, kind of like there was a lot more to that evening than I knew. "Your lungs had collapsed. We had to move fast. We had to put you under to do what we had to do to keep you breathing. It was not a pretty site trying to get you down right away. You put up quite a struggle, and I hoped that you did not remember much of what happened. We had to get pretty physical, and another nurse told me that you wouldn't remember the events of that day. We had to set you up with a breathing machine. I had never worked with this procedure before, so I didn't know its effects. I didn't believe the other nurse when she said that you would not remember anything, but I am relieved to hear it from you."

7
You Only Need One Kidney

I learned that today upward of eleven million Americans unknowingly are affected by some form of kidney disease. Of that number 230,000 are treated yearly for some form of kidney failure. Recent statistics also revealed that the kidney is now the number One sought after human organ for transplantation in these United States.

It is embarrassing for me to admit that, before I got sick with this disease, I knew absolutely nothing about it. I was one of those people who did not get involved in other people's business. The cancers, the diabetes, the strokes, the aids, and heart attack victims, and all other health unfortunates lived across the street and down the road from me. They were featured in the papers, and made their guest appearances on the five o'clock news. I did very little to champion their causes. I supported their organization with a monetary donation here and there, but not much else.

When one has been as fortunate as I throughout their lifetime, the last thing on one's mind is to expect a visit from the angel of misfortune. The fact is that God has protected my family and me from misfortunes over many years. I refuse to believe that this single experience means that He has stopped having favor with me.

The experience is life changing in more ways than one. Besides the physical alteration, I have had to stop and prioritize the events of my life. Like Job in the Bible I feel responsible to persevere in my faith and look for the opportunity to be instrumental in doing God's work.   It took a while for me to come to grips with myself and accept these conditions that add new limitations to my body.   Like my son who asked, "What did this family ever do to God that was so awful, that God should punish us this way, similarly I asked myself, "Why me Lord."   I don't want to accept the fact that I am an ESRD, End Stage Renal Disease patient.   Even the name sounds like something pretty awful, something contagious, or maybe even as the name implies, something final.

My son, Armando, presumed like I did that we had the control of our destiny in our hands. I could see that he had difficulty believing that his Dad was in such a disabling condition.   He looked around the dialysis center and immediately asked me, "Well, Dad what's the next move"? What do we do to get the ball rolling for this transplant business?" He expected me to have an answer for him. He could not see a problem, not if this was about a kidney. His response was, "Dad you have five kids, that's a total of (10) ten kidneys, and you only need one." I remember having mumbled something about waiting awhile. The fact was that I didn't know any more than he did what the next step was, but I had the feeling that it wasn't going to be standard operating procedure. Nothing in my life ever is, and I don't see any reason why this should change now.

Jorge Joseph Taylor

I kept expecting to be awakened. I just could not bring myself to believe that this was occurring to me. It was such an unbelievable experience. I just knew that I would be wakened at any time soon. One day I was fine, and the next day my world had been turned inside out. I am flat on my back most of the time. I have my entire family in turmoil, and my friends are bewildered and just stare at me with the saddest expressions on their faces. I could not in my wildest dream imagine how I got here.

I left the hospital two weeks later with hypertension and kidney disease. As an end stage renal patient, I am now dependent on dialysis for the rest of my natural life, unless I undergo a kidney transplant. It all happened with unbelievable speed. Most of my hospital stay was under sedation. While in the hospital I was dialyzed, but it didn't hit me that after leaving the hospital I would be immediately attending some clinic every other day on an outpatient basis.

The seriousness of this disease did not leave its impression until I realized that I can not stop going to the clinic. I can't get tired and not go. I can't even get sick and stay home in bed, on the day that I'm to dialyze. I can't just get into my truck and retreat into the mountains for a few days without regard to the day of the week and planning my dialysis in advance.

This past summer the temperature outside rose to a sizzling 95 plus degrees in much of these United States and stayed there for the better part of the summer. For many of those days I wanted to take a dip in somebody's refreshing pool, but because of my catheter I was not able. The catheter restricted my activities tremendously for fear of infections. Another restriction is my fluid intake. I just can't have a nice long cold drink in the middle of a sizzling summer day like most normal people do to satisfy and quench the thirst inside; at least not without knowing how much fluid I have already had. On the average we are allowed a kilo of flied daily, and I could have already reached my limitation for the day, regardless of what the thermostat reads outside.

Part II

Memoir
The Process
03/09/01

I can't believe that it has already been a year since I started coming to this *dialysis* center. A year is not a very long time, yet some how it seems like a life time to me. I know one thing. I am ready to be through with this love-hate relationship that this machine and I have established. Every other day for the past year, I've had a rendezvous with a dialysis machine, which last, for four long hours. Some people have had a long term 20 years-plus relationship with these machines.

I have seen patients go to sleep for a good portion of their four hours dialysis ride, and even consume a full meal while they are dialyzing. I am still a novice at this. I don't know that I can do neither. It just doesn't seem appropriate. It could be that I am afraid of being caught asleep when those unbearable cramps decide to take me hostage. I have noticed quite a few patients cramping. It appears to be a side effect of this treatment.

Hemodialysis seems to be the treatment of choice. It is a procedure that utilizes a dialysis machine to remove the blood, along with its impurities, from the body. Once the blood has been removed, it then passes through a filter that traps the poisons and returns the purified blood back to the body. In essence, the Hemodialysis machine is a man-made kidney that functions outside the body. The treatment or time the patient spends on the machine is referred to as a *run* or a *ride*. When a ride goes well and there is no abnormality to report, it is documented as *uneventful.* The machine continuously monitors blood pressure, heart rate, pulse, oxygen levels, intravenous medications and other measurements.

The machine connects to the arm via a hypodermic needles and an *Access.* There are two types of A*ccesses:* *the Fistula type* and the *Graph.* Two hypodermic needles are commonly placed in either type of A*ccess.* The *Fistula* utilizes ones own veins and arteries to form the access beneath the skin while the *Graph* is formed by utilizing a man-made material to do the same.

Under normal circumstances, the patient has an appointment time at the clinic or hospital. The patient then washes his or her hands, access area and weighs themselves prior to taking a seat and starting the dialysis run.

The option to Hemodialysis is *Peritoneal Dialysis or PD.* There are two different procedures available for patients who chose *peritoneal dialysis. T*hey are as follow: *Continuous Ambulatory Peritoneal Dialysis or CAPD,* and *Continuous Cycling Peritoneal Dialysis or CCPD.* In either case, fluid is introduced into the peritoneal lining of the abdomen where it remains for a designated period of time. During this time the body uses a process called *osmosis* to extract the impurities from the blood.

The patient then performs what are called *exchanges* to remove the contaminated fluid from the peritoneal cavity replace it with clean fluid, and repeat the process all over again.

Differences between *CAPD* and *CCPD*

CAPD is a series of applications administered through out the day depending on the doctor's prescribed dosage. The doctor will prescribe the number of *exchanges* and their interval. In the comfort of their home the patient is responsible for replacing contaminated fluids with clean fluid.

CCPD, unlike the *CAPD,* is administered in a single application. It is administered mostly at night while the patient is asleep. The duration of this application is from eight to ten hours every night. A machine is employed and programmed to keep track of the intake and amount of fluid, the time it stays in the peritoneal, as well as, exchange times.

Transplant is of course the closest option to the operation of an original kidney function. This treatment option requires that patients meet eligibility requirements before becoming candidates for *transplant.*

It is my understanding that every chronic *dialysis* patient should qualify as a *transplant candidate.* The criterion for a *transplant candidate* is that his or her kidney function be diminished to less than fifteen per cent of capacity. The patient must be in need of *dialysis* or a *transplant* in order to maintain life. Even though all the patients that I know probably fall under these circumstances, they must still be screened and pass a *clinical criteria*. The *clinical criteria* pretty much contradicts the fact that this individual must be sick unto death and that without the administration of either H*emodialysis* or a *transplant* this individual will die.

The *clinical criteria* are that the patient must have a stable heart and lung function, be free of infectious diseases, and must be highly motivated toward a strict regiment of medication.

The *transplant* program identifies two types of donors. *Living Donors* and the *Cadaver Donors.* The living donors can either be a related or unrelated individual. If a match to the recipient blood and tissue type cannot be found in the living donor's category then the recipient will be placed on the National Cadaver donor's list.

Hemodialysis is the most common of all options available now.

The purpose of the dialysis machine is to perform some of the duties that healthy kidneys do. It cleans the blood by extracting toxins and excess fluids accumulating in the body. In essence this machine is a man made kidney that functions outside the body during the period of time that one is attached to it.

Memoir
Man's best Friend
03/10/01

In the previous chapter, I wrote that I was ready to terminate the love-hate relationship that has developed between the dialysis machine and me. I must confess my ignorance, my childish emotional passion of anger and a lack of patience. Who am I to question the hands of God the potter? Who am I to know the extent of His mind and His plans? Well, had my kidneys failed in 1942 such an option would have been irrelevant or better yet non-existent. You see the dialysis machine did not come about until 1943 by W. J. Kolff and H. Berk from the Netherlands.

So what happened to *ESRD* patients before Kolff invented the *dialysis machine* in 1943? Apparently, the advances of technology did not address that question. The designation *end stage renal disease* had a more applicable significance. The patient would die from the accumulation of toxins produced by his or her own body.

Dialysis has come a long way and it has quite a team of individuals contributing to its development to thank for it.

The term *"dialysis"* is attributed to the chemist, Professor Thomas Graham in 1861. During an experiment, he noticed that the diffusion of crystalloids was possible through vegetable parchment, and so he named the process *dialysis*.

In 1913 ,the first *hemodialysis* procedure was performed by a group of individuals including Abel, Roundtree, and Turner to establish the first artificial kidney.

It was only experimental at this point. Only the use of animal blood was extracted and successfully returned to the animal.

Other advances were made during the century, but the most notable was by the German George Haas who performed the first successful human *haemodialysis* in 1924. The procedure only lasted a total of fifteen minutes, but it set the stage for that love-hate relationship that has existed now for almost eighty years.

The dialysis machine itself has seen quite a transformation in size, looks and capabilities.

Its development went from a huge rotating drum by Kolff in 1943, to the tubing wound around a vertically mounted screen in the 1950s by Nils Alwall, to the Kolff-Bringham dialyser in the same period. At one time, they even modified and utilized a washing machine to dialyze. I am sure that as long as individual's kidneys fail the need for dialyzing will continue to invent a better replacement for the kidney.

Memoir
Choosing to Stay
03/11/01

During my first six months at the clinic for dialysis treatment, I dared not fall asleep during my ride for fear of getting caught off guard by a cramp attack on my lower back. Cramping on my legs and arms I could withstand, but pain in my lower back was out of the question. To date, I have yet to see another patient who cramps in his or her lower back. What I felt was a pulsating sensation. It came in waves and got stronger with each pulsating sensation until it reached its peak where the pressure is strongest. It then worked its way back down and decreased until it subsided. I try my best to keep these cramps from getting started, because once they start, they continue pulsating until they peak. Cramping elsewhere in the body could be alleviated with about 100 ccs of saline administered intravenously.

I have often wondered about the story behind each of these faces here at the dialysis center. They seem to reflect a resignation after much struggle and resistance to their circumstances. A coming to grips with the imperfections that life offers us on a personal level. I remember a nurse once telling me that I still have a choice. I do not have to accept to live in my present condition. I can totally avoid the discomfort of dialyzing, but that choice too has its consequences.

Sitting next to me is a patient who comes in at his appointed time with a pair of prosthetics not just one but two of them. While he is in the chair dialyzing, his metal legs are leaning up against the wall. The pain that we experience must indeed be a relative thing. This is indeed a fighter. I have something in common with everybody in this clinic. We are all here because our bodies are lacking the efficient function of their kidneys. We all can at least understand that we cannot depend on ourselves to continue to support our existence. Some of us have more critical illnesses like diabetes that tend to complicate things. The point is that after looking around and witnessing these people in their circumstances, I'm filled with shame when I find myself absorbed in complaisance.

Memoir
Moving On
03/12/01

I have not cramped now for a few days. This is good. Just because I haven't doesn't mean that someone else isn't cramping. The clinic that I go to has approximately 20 chairs and operates from 6 a.m. to 10 p.m. It is considered a fairly large clinic. The environment at the clinic is rather unpredictable. Sometimes you see folks getting dialyzed and are never seen again. They are called visitors. They are actually traveling or passing through and made arrangements to get their blood serviced at this facility. The facility sometimes has a transient hotel type environment. That appearance is even more prominent when your schedule happens to change from Mondays, Wednesdays, Fridays, to Tuesdays, Thursdays, Saturday. You now become a transient at your own center.

Speaking of being a visitor, I am traveling to Warrenton North Carolina to visit with my father in law. My wife's father has been relentless in his own confrontation with cancer for some time now. We are going to visit him and encourage his effort over the weekend. I have made arrangement, to dialyze there during my stay. I am a bit leery about scheduling this appointment there. I realize that it is very convenient to be able to dialyze nationally however, I am a bit nervous about dialyzing elsewhere.

I found out today that Ted, a handsome brother and very pleasant man, passed away. I had not seen him for a couple of weeks. The food that his wife brought him while he dialyzed left its aroma all through the clinic. Sometimes it was fish and other times it was fried chicken. There was another patient that passed away that same week, but I did not know her very well. Ted had been having a rough go at it, after he fell and broke his hip. The tech that shared this news with me felt that Ted may be better off. At the very least, he won't be in any pain at all.

I have witnessed a few patients move on to meet their maker, and it becomes a sad time for all of us at the center, including the professionals. I suppose that it is not much different than the family that I have fostered at work. A certain amount of bonding has taken place.

One of the technicians was explaining to me that she was glad that this incident occurred on her day off, because she couldn't watch another one of her patient, die. She said that the last time this happened to her, she had just returned from lunch to find one of her patients deceased. She said that she could not stop crying for the rest of the day.

Memoir
Captain Marvel

My mother had packed up most of the dishes and clothing in crates lined up against the wall in our two-room apartment back in the old country. The mahogany china closet stood empty up against the walls. The beautiful matching table with its two center leaves removed stood in the middle of the room with only a table-cloth to protect it.

Excitement jumped from my two sisters to me. We just couldn't contain it. It was like the night before the first day of school. I'm sure you remember how difficult it was to fall a-sleep that night.

The sheer anticipation of a new experience, new friends, new teachers and a complete new set of circumstances, what a rush! Yes! That is how we felt except that this wasn't a new school; it wasn't just a new neighborhood and friends to play with; it was an entirely new country. It was the revolution of a culture shock.

Mom was selling everything to begin a new life in the United States of America. It was our new beginning. Somewhere between our night time chatter and mom's reprimands the sandman came calling. It was the voice of the lady in distress that prompted me into action. Immediately I stood up at the edge of the bed and proclaiming the magical words Sha Zam. A loud boom followed, and I found myself transformed into my Captain Marvel Super hero costume. I stood up at the edge of the bed and took a standing leap into the air.

I landed stomach first onto my mother's mahogany table, slid on the tablecloth right off the polished table and landed in a wash bucket packed with china sitting in a corner of the room.

Needless to say, that the crashing into the washtub full of mom's china woke me up. I don't know what possessed me to retrieve information archived so long ago. I was just a young boy, with no care in the world, except my dreams. Maybe these thoughts are appropriate for times like these when soaring with eagles seems to be relegated to dreams of our past.

Memoir
On Traveling
03/14/01

I have been thinking about my wife. I don't feel her being very happy these days. I can't help from thinking that my renal condition has been contributing to her low spirits. One of the realities that we are faced with is travel restrictions. It was apparent to me that there would be changes in our travel habits, even though I was constantly reminded that this disease will not restrict my travel habits.

In previous years, my wife's boutique business required us to travel to New York, Dallas, and California's garment districts once or twice a year. Besides the steady business trips, our vacation trips to Puerto Vallarta and Jamaica had simply just stopped. Since the onset of this kidney disease, traveling has been curtailed.

My wife's dad's health took a turn for the worse, and she decided to go visit him. This will be her second trip to her home town in Warrenton. She asked me to go with her to visit her dad who was engaged in a noble struggle against cancer.

It would be good for me to take this trip. Her Father and I made and shared good memories in New York and in North Carolina. I'm anxious to see him now, or maybe I am confusing this with the anxiety and pain that reflects from my wife's eyes.

I can see how spouses are affected by this disease and suffer the pains and discomfort right along with their husbands or wives. Some spouses unable to provide a change in the circumstances of their better half, will come and sit with their spouses through out the entire duration of their haemodialysis treatment.

I am very curious about my experience at a different center. I will be able to compare their services and bring you back a report. I am about three hours into my treatment, and cramping normally occurs going into my last hour. I must put this computer away so that I can be ready to react. Normally when cramping begins I scramble to my feet. I feel like I have a little control when I am on my feet.

Memoir
Listening to my Body
03/16/01

Jorge Joseph Taylor

Last Sunday my friend Jim Wheeler mentioned that he thought I was putting on some weight. I wanted to believe him. This week everyone recognizes that there is some abnormality about my appearance. I usually wear a size 141/2 inches neck size shirt, but today I am wearing a size 16 ½ size shirt.

I thought that this was a result of some salty Chinese food that I had eaten the night before. Some of the nurses at the center just knew that I had blown the fluid restriction, of my diet.

I noticed that after dialysis the swelling in my face seems to have gone down some. The next time I went to dialysis the doctor was there. He did not like what he saw. He referred me to the hospital the very next day for a picture of my chest that quickly revealed that my arteries were blocked. The hospital staff placed a stint in my chest. The pressure was alleviated, and the swelling soon went down.

I must confess to you that being aware of my body nuances has not been my strongest suit. After this episode, however; I will do my best to be more aware of feelings that are occurring constantly in my body. Being ignorant of the volatility in my body is probably one of the reasons that I am in this position.

I am normally not a person that abuses my fluids. In fact, I am very seldom two kilos over my dry weight. This should have given me some indication that my fluid was not the problem. I have been noticing that there are many professionals and technicians who assume that the patient is ignorant about this disease and his treatment. They do not hesitate for one minute to lay blame on a patient who has no knowledge of his circumstances.

I have also noticed that the reverse to this principle is also true. The more knowledge a patient posses in their defense, the more respect seems to come their way. I have decided to dedicate myself to becoming a model dialysis patient. I will learn as much as I can about this disease that I have. I will learn as much as there is to know about the treatments available to me, and I will continue to discover the ways in which my body works.

Memoir
Southern Style Dialysis
03/19/01

Well, I am sitting in the chair at Gambro Medical Center in Henderson, North Carolina. This is my first experience outside of my home center. The facility is rather large. It outgrew its previous location and added space for an additional 12 chairs in another part of this building. Between both locations in this facility there are a total of 32 chairs.

Niki is one of the nurses on this shift. She was not only a professional in her knowledge and demeanor, but the sincerity and kindness of her bedside manner was enough to dispel any discomfort. I immediately thought of that southern hospitality. After all, this was the south. After mentioning that to Niki , she reminded me that she would hope that her own patient, are treated the way that she treats others visiting with her center. I observed her techniques as we conversed. I watched her change my dressing. She used alcohol and iodine to clean and disinfect. She explained that the alcohol removes the sticky gummy substance left behind by the silk tape, and then the iodine kills the bacteria that may be growing around the perm catheter area.

"I don't take any chances, and I do believe in iodine," was Niki's response to the reason for the procedure. I watched the other patients in my vicinity, and they all seemed to be if not content with their treatment, at least satisfied.

The facility was laid out in a horse shoe shape, making it possible for everyone to have visual contact with everyone else; most importantly it was somewhat convenient for the health professionals to monitor all the patients by just turning around in the same bay. The dialysis machines were somewhat different to what I am used to. The functionality and basic appearance were similar.

The nutritionist name is Tammy. She unveiled a technique associated with helping the patient familiarize themselves with their phosphorus. The name of the game was appropriately called Phosphorus Bingo and Black Out. This was a fantastic game. Not everybody played, but the bay became alive as Tammy Sanford called out the name of foods to be found on the bingo card that were high in phosphorus.

Memoir
A Failed Kidney-God's Gift
03/28/01

When my family realized that I had indeed lost the function of my kidneys and were aware that a kidney transplant was the closest thing to having your own kidney, they began pushing me to inquire about a kidney transplant. The doctor informed me that he would recommend me for a transplant only after I have had a diagnosis of the mass that was found on my left kidney.

The mass on my kidney was discovered while investigating a malfunctioning kidney. Diagnosis was inconclusive. To make a long story short, my doctor would not recommend me for a transplant until the mass was diagnosed conclusively to be a non-malignant growth. The result came back, and the growth was malignant. I could not wait for the result of this test. I was so certain that it would be negative. Now the transplant goes out the window for at least two years down the road.

Everyone is now adopting the idea that I have been extremely lucky to have a failed kidney.

My Urologists explained that if my kidneys had not failed they would not have discovered the cancer growth until it had spread to other parts of my body. So the verdict from my doctor is that now I must wait two years and be found free of any additional growth before he can recommend me for a transplant.

I could see the disappointment in my son Armando's face when I shared this information with him. My impatient son, a product of today's instant gratification instant microwave fixes, had a lump in his throat. I did not let him know that I had a lump larger than his that I forced myself to swallow. I wanted to apologize to him and my wife and my other, sons and daughters for dragging them through this. If only I could get through this quickly maybe they wouldn't realize how bad of a trip this would turn out to be. There must be something here that my Lord wants me to learn. Maybe I have to pay some dues.

I feel as if I have traveled to a very desolate place, somewhere towards the vicinity of the edge of my world. It was a place that I did not recognize. My heart bled for the people that I found there. They were like the clowns at the circus whose external smiles and laughter hid the heart broken feelings beneath their skin. I penetrated the very stage of their existence, and saw the reality that they lived with daily. Their reality was being poked with needles every other day. I felt their aches and pains of cramping as a result of their dialysis treatment. I saw the devastation in the expressionless eyes of diabetic patient. I learned what it is like to coexist with that silent killer hyper tension.

This is a very peculiar world. It reminds me of the television episode "Survivor". We have to learn about the foods that are edible. All that is good to make a normal person healthy is not allowed to the renal patient. Watching our fluid intake has become a ritualistic practice. I use to hear my doctor and others preach about 6 to eight glasses of water per day. Well in this world you can forget that.

Jorge Joseph Taylor

What is recommended is a juice glass or coffee cup half full of water, or maybe a cup of ice chips and the words "watch your fluid intake" has become a coined phrase that you are expected to wear on your forehead always.

Memoir
An Ounce of Prevention
03/29/01

Jorge Joseph Taylor

Today has been a good day. Dr. Block came by to see me as he does once a month to share information of my labs and to see how I'm doing in general. The conversation was light with a few jokes here and there. My laboratory report was very good.   The Doctor had to hold my epogen medication due to the increase production level of my red blood cells. "It is not something you have to worry about Jorge. Your red blood cells appear to be as healthy as my own. Jorge when did you have that operation to remove the cancer growth. Has it been a year yet?"

"No Doc", I replied. "It was sometime in July." The Doctor didn't reveal all that he had in his mind, but I had the feeling that it was of a positive nature. "Why don't you make an appointment to go next month?" I nodded my head in reply. He knew that I needed that early vote of confident from him.

When I think about how this could have been prevented, Jennie comes to mind. She reminds me that all the signs were there. She is absolutely right. I recall the mountain trip that we took with friends. My friend bought several bags of pork skins that we all enjoyed without a care or concern.   I remember seeing spots momentarily while driving up the mountain. During another trip, this time to New York the same thing happened. I chose to ignore these warning signs. Then there were the episodes of headaches that followed. I did not ignore them.   I tried to treat them by using some over the counter medications

80

that seems to work in the beginning. This was a sure sign because I rarely get headaches.

One day at work the pain was so excruciating that it drove me to a fetal position under my desk. These pains magnified themselves both in frequency and intensity. It is imperative that we listen to what our body is saying to us. This was the way to prevention. This is where the cost is minimal. The pain is less and lives are extended.

It is important to realize that by the time you start to feel symptoms you have already incurred substantial damage to your kidneys. So how do we combat this decease or can we do anything about it. Here is what my nephrologists say on this topic.

"Prevention and education in this area are extremely important and necessary. One of the first things that people think of, is their diet. To some degree we can look to diet, but not in the case of a hereditary decease. Whether prevention can be found in our diet or whether it is something hereditary, we do not know. We have yet to find the answers, and that is why there are research programs like the one that I am involved in. Although we have learned quite a bit about the kidney and its function, there is still quite a bit to uncover, but we will find out the answers to why kidneys fail."

There are a few things that we do know about kidney disease: It is hereditary. If a member of your family has had kidney failure, then this would be a good reason for you to insist that your doctor performs the necessary test to determine the health of your kidneys. High blood pressure is a disease that in most cases is the fore runner to kidney failure. Again if you or any member of your family suffers from hypertension, you could be a candidate for renal failure without knowing it. Diabetes is the other disease that is closely associated with renal failure.

Prevention is really going to start with what feeling good feels like. You have got to learn to know your body. Know a little history of your family for your own protection and well being, what you learn could save your life. Education is what is going to erase our ignorance of this disease. We need to become aggressive and involved in our treatment.

Memoir
From The Edge
04/11/01

The Nurse asked me,"What are we doing about your access," Maybe I should explain what she meant by that. When one loses the function of their kidneys and becomes a renal patient that relies on the use of a dialysis machine, an emergency access called a perm catheter is placed on the patient's body. This perm catheter is the place where the dialysis machine connects to the blood flow, (arteries and vines). It has been over a year now since this perm catheter has been installed.

The name perm catheter is deceiving because it is made up of two words, permanent and catheter. This installation is not of a permanent nature as the name implies. The procedure is only in place until a graft or a fistula is installed.

Most patients receive a perm catheter that is used for approximately six month. During this time the more permanent access is installed, and usage begins somewhere within 6 months of installation. Needless to tell you that the word normal does not abide with me, so this does not apply. I did go to day surgery and I had the fistula installed in my upper left arm. Technicians and nurses can feel and hear the thrill (a sensation of the blood rushing through vein easy enough), but when it comes time to stick it with the needle it's a different story. Try as they may, they cannot seem to find it.

The result of a cat scan reported that the fistula is embedded too deep in my arm, and access is very difficult if at all possible. We can't even go back to the surgeon that performed the initial operation to fix the problem. The doctor that did the work is no longer around. So we must find a different surgeon to first see if this procedure can be saved by lifting the fistula closer to the surface. Until then we continue the use of my perm catheter.

Any nephrologists would confirm that a kidney patient is challenged by far too many incidents from those that maybe predictable side effects to surprises that this disease is revealing to date. Professionals are just now learning that perm catheter left in the chest for a prolong period can cause more damage than good by shrinking or collapsing the veins resulting in blockage.

It has become difficult for me to abuse my fluids intake since two kilos of fluids is enough to cause swelling in my face and neck. Most mornings I can't leave the house until drainage occurs in my face and this may take a couple of hours.

Memoir
A Farewell letter
04/18/01

April 15, 2001 Is important to most people in the U.S. because it is also know as tax date , but I'm thinking about it because that was the date that Gary Hamilton left us to relocate in Arizona. Who is Gary Hamilton? I am so glad that you asked that question. He was the Lowry Dialysis Facility Administrator. Gary kept things running smooth in the clinic. He manages the entire staff of nurses, technicians and office help. He maintains the equipment in the facility. The appearance of the facility gives an impression to visitors and new patients too. Last but certainly not least is Gary's demeanor. His demeanor is important because when he communicates to his facility his demeanor helps to carry his message. I have only been a patient for little more than a year but I have seen the different effect that a dialysis facility can have on patients.

In a letter dated April 10, Gary explained why he was moving away to Arizona. This is one of the most beautiful letters I have ever read I contacted Gary and asked him if he minded if I shared it with you. So the following is that letter.

To all of my patients:

As you may have heard, I am moving to Arizona. If I have not spent much time with you, or had a chance to explain what has prompted my decision to move, please forgive me. This has been one of the hardest things I have ever had to do. I am leaving a great family of patient and staff. Then why leave?

About two months ago now my oldest son Brandon called me on a Friday afternoon and told me he was going to the prom, and could I teach him how to tie a tie. After teaching him how to tie it over the phone, I hung up the phone and started to cry. Brandon is almost 15 years old now I have been away for almost 10 years. Dads are supposed to be there for their children and I am not. Their mother is a great person and has done a great job raising them, but now as they become young men, I owe it to them to try and instill in them the same values that my father instilled in me.

The main reason that I'm writing you instead of sitting with each of you individually is because I don't feel I am emotionally strong enough right now. I have given all I have to try and create an environment where all of my patients feel safe and well cared for; an environment that the staff wants to come to work and care for my patients, and a feeling of family. I can only hope that you, the most important part of our center, an the reason I get up in the morning feel that I have been reasonably successful in accomplishing our goals, and most importantly, know that I truly care about each and everyone of you.

I wish you all the very best

Memoir
Ronnie
05/14/01

Ron is a new patient. He seems to have taken to me. It is only about his third treatment. The first time I saw him, he seems to have been cramping and having a very difficult time with his treatment.   It wasn't long after that he began to entrust me with personal information regarding his renal condition.

Ron is a young white male approximately 30 years old with a very lean built. He moves swiftly and deliberate unlike most of the patients in the clinic, whose movements can be very slow and sluggish, especially at the end of their treatment.

Ron has upward of 12 operations that started when he was a child. At the age of 15 he was subject to an operation that removed his left kidney. Lately his other kidney had not been doing a good job cleaning his blood, so the Dr. decided that he should begin to dialyze. He showed me his arms and explained that the numerous scars are as the result from the attempt to find good enough veins to install a graph." None would work for me", he said. The more Ron and I talked the more his circumstances seem to be like my own. Like Me Ron must be dialyzed through the catheter in his chest because our veins are too thin to allow a more acceptable means of dialysis. This makes us more prone to infections from the open access in our chest. It also prevents us from being able to submerge in water. So although showers are possible under the most cautious care, a dip in the pool during summer or any other time for that matter is totally out of the question. The Doctor was concerned with Ron's work ethics. He delivers Pizza with one of the local Pizza parlor's in the evenings then at the crack of dawn he is up delivering milk. Ron just has no demeanor of an end stage renal patient, then again who really knows what is the looks or demeanor of an end stage renal individual.

Memoir
A Prayer Warrior
05/19/01

There is time on my hands to think. Now there is, only because God listened to your prayers and petitions. He decided to grant your requests. Time does not belong to anyone but God. He gives it, and He takes it away. I believe this with all my heart. If you don't believe me just ask any of my prayer warrior friends who spent endless hours asking God to grant me more time, and not take me just yet.

I think about what is really important now. I think about the time that I have spent just spinning my wheels, chasing after the wind and squandering the time that God entrusted me with. My trip to the edge brought me face to face with that place where time ends, and things are not retrievable. My trip to the edge brought me to that door that opens outward into another dimension, Eternity.

I began a journey to eternity that lasted only for a moment. I left my body for a minute, and on my way out the door my passage was rejected. I can't say much about eternity, because God kept time on my side.

I could discern the presence of my prayer warrior's spirit. I knew that their spirit remained in constant communication with God, on my behalf. God answered them positively, just like he had done with Isaiah on behalf of King Hezekiah, when He granted him fifteen more years to complete his task here in time.

King Hezekiah was sick unto death. God had told him to get his house in order, because he was very sick and about to die. King Hezekiah prayed to God. God reversed His decision and extended the life of the King. Read Isaiah Ch. 38.

I did make a promise to God that if He allowed me more time as He did King Hezekiah, I would spend it in a more productive manner, helping his people and glorifying his name.

Only God is really aware of all the true members of the team of prayer warriors who communicate with him daily. Among His faithful prayer warriors is Mrs. Sheila Barnes. She reminded me daily of her prayers. While I recovered at home not a single day went by that my prayer warrior did not call me to pray with me concerned about my health and to let me know that she was constantly in touch with God petitioning for my recovery. I know that you haven't asked but if you did ask for some advice I would tell you that not withstanding other elements of survival, a prayer warrior is an indispensable tool to have in your survival kit. I cannot stress the importance of a prayer warrior. This is a must have.

Where do you go to find a prayer warrior? As for myself, I'm blessed. I have a prayer warrior right here in my family. All my children know who God is. For this I am eternally thankful. My youngest son, Miguel, however, is the prayer warrior in my family. I have never doubted that I am continuously being lifted up by him in prayer. A prayer warrior is an individual who specializes in spiritual matters. It is one who knows how to reach God and communicate with God. They can be found most likely in the membership of a Bible believing Christian church.

Among the first century Christians, the Apostle James would be my choice as the closest thing to a prayer warrior. This is not to say that the contribution of the others was not essential to the well being of the entire body of Christ. It's just that prayer warriors are special.

Memoir
Dreams And Visions
05/20/01

I am not bubbling with energy today. This is a strange sickness. Sometimes it does not appear as I am sick. Other times my mind has difficulty instructing the rest of my body parts. In my family, we always try to support any member engaged in attaining a goal. Tonight my lovely wife, the Rev. Jennie Taylor, is scheduled to preach her first sermon at our church's Wednesday night mid-week services. It is unfortunate that I am not able to support her this time. I think that knowing this is making me even sicker. I must try to engage a more positive thought.

Dreams have always played a very impressionable role in my life, ever since I was a child. As a child, most dreams I really tried not to remember. I would push them back in my mind as far back as I could send them. Most of the dreams bordered on horror and night mare. You can see why I never gave them much credence. However, now that I am an adult I try to find more understanding in the things of life, I find myself searching my bible. It talks about young men and vision and old men dreaming. It mentions God talking to humans through the medium, and the interpretation of dreams.

Why am I telling you all this about dreams? Well, when I was in the hospital in route to the edge, I experienced many dreams most of them are beyond my ability to express. One of them I recall seems to have had a theme or motto. My entire family was at the hospital.

I had just awakened. The sedatives they had given me still had some influence on me. There seemed to have been much confusion and crying in the room, but not withstanding all of this, my spirit was not disturbed.

In my dreams, I had seen the reality of the hospital room that was rather old, in need of upkeep and refurbishment. Somewhere on the continuum of dreams and visions I saw another room that was freshly painted with bright colors and a modern décor. I was a product of both pictures. In the prior I was actually bedridden, and the picture was in black and white. In the second picture was that of a completely refurbished environment and my health was better I was able to walk. Bishop Phillips and his wife La Quila where visiting me, at the time. I turned to the Bishop and asked him, "What was the meaning of such a dream?" In a very quiet tone but with a deliberate emphasis, the Bishop interpreted my dream, only he called it a vision or a revelation.

The two pictures he said were to be regarded as a transition from my present circumstances to a vision and revelation of a continued, but refurbished and renewed life.

This was the answer to the prayers of the many. It was a continuation from the old black and white to a drastically improved refurbished and renewed life. This dream was not like the others that deserved to be buried in the deepest part of one's mind. This one was different.

Jorge Joseph Taylor

This was a good dream. This was one of those dreams where you win the lotto, and you wake up looking for the money. You know the one!

Initially, there was misunderstanding on my part, but I never ceased to reassure and comfort my family around me that the will of God will prevail.

Memoir
The Transplant List
6/22/01

Jorge Joseph Taylor

I saw Ronnie today. He had some bitter sweet news to tell me. I had not seen Ronnie for a few weeks now.   He always shows up with a smile on his face and an attitude that transforms any gloomy day into one to be thankful for.

Anyway Ron shared with me that he had been to the hospital to get a new perm catheter, installed in his chest. The former one had malfunctioned. Without elaborating much about the malfunctioning perm catheter, Ron began telling me that he had been placed on the list, the kidney transplant list.

Ronnie is an energetic young man. I don't think he has an ounce of fat on his body. He told me that he had a pizza delivery job that keeps him going until about 10 o'clock at night, but that's not enough for Ronnie. The energizer bunny does not have anything on him. He has to go get a second job as a milk man. So he gets up at 4 o'clock in the morning to deliver milk.

I was as happy to hear the news as Ron was to tell it. Just to think of the possibility of being quote unquote normal again. Not having to cramp every other day would be a thing of the past. Not having to worry about your fluid intake.   Not having to plan trips around a dialysis center. Not having to worry about a pulmonary edema. Not to worry about your phosphorous, your potassium, your calcium and other chemistry observation performed monthly. In my case, not having to worry about my face looking like an ugly fruit in the mornings. This is just a few factors that may reduce the stress for a renal patient.

Ronnie received the ultimate news any renal patient would want to hear. He asked me about my own transplant status. I explained to Ronnie that due to my recent episode with cancer, I had to wait two to five years before I could be eligible for a transplant. To date, a year has already passed, so my wait is down to one year before I can be placed on the kidney transplant list.

It is my observation that a kidney transplant is the closest option for a restored quality of life. It is amazing that not all renal patients will select that option for varied reason. There is a level of commitment involved in continued medication that must be observed. Likewise, if commitment is not adhered to, the risk factor concerning rejection can be fatal.

My God exposed me to this reality even before I lost the use of my kidneys. During a conversation with my plumber, whom I trusted with all my plumbing needs, he explained that he couldn't finish a job that he started, because he had to go to dialysis. At the time, I did not know what dialysis was, so he explained to me that he had lost the use of his kidneys. That summer Lamont, my plumber, told me that he would be going in for a transplant shortly. That was the last time that I talked to Lamont. I heard that he had died because of some trouble with the transplant. So there are risks associated with the transplant of a kidney. After weighing the risks and examining the options available, some people would rather stay with the familiar grounds of dialysis, rather than to venture out into uncharted waters of a transplant.

My wife shared a conversation with me that she had with her banker friend. They communicated about the common challenges we face concerning this renal problem. To her surprise, the lady banker confessed to having similar challenges with her husband. The lady banker explained to my wife that they had tried the transplant way. The health related set backs were so many and complex that they resigned themselves to continue the more familiar process of dialyzing every other day. She said that they know the challenges and risks they face in the familiar grounds of the dialysis environment.

Other patients may not be candidates for kidney transplant because of an age, or health factor. Who is to say that one should continue with dialysis or opt for the more radical choice of a life sustaining transplant? There is no blue print to follow here. All there is are consequences to our choices. Even though we can learn from the circumstances and decisions of others, to consider choosing without the input of our own circumstances is probably the riskiest position to be in.

Memoir
Fistula or Graph
06/27/01

I stopped believing a physician or a nurse that tells me this is really a simple procedure.

I have come to learn that no procedure with me is simple. When such things as drawing blood require the attempt of two or three technicians, the head nurse, and ultimately the doctor, then we have progressed past simple.

The dialysis center's head nurse scheduled me for a surgical procedure to implant a Fistula. The fistula is one of the choices used to create an access. The other possibility is called a Graph.

The Fistula or Graph unites a prominent vein and an artery. This procedure, when successful, will create an access in the arm or legs that allows dialysis to take place. After the procedures it takes approximately three to six months for the Fistula to mature enough to be stuck with a hypodermic needle. I have had to go back for a venal graph. The venal graph is basically an x-ray that reveals the position and condition of the veins inside one's body.

My venal graph showed that my fistula is buried too deep into my arm, and unable to be successfully stuck with a hypodermic needle. Here I am, a year after the simple procedure, we are at a crossroad having to decide again to go back in and untie the procedure.

Besides the function of dialyzing my blood, the Fistula or Graph buries the access under your skin, hiding the access from plain view, and protecting the body by limiting the possibility of contamination from infection. This mode of dialyzing first and foremost gets the job done; secondly, it acts as a prevention against infections. The last benefit that I see is it allows the patient the privilege to function in his environment as normal as he once did. Not only are we trying to look normal, but we are trying to do the things that normal people do.

The difference between a graph and a fistula is its component and durability. In the case of the graph the part used to join the artery and the vein is a plastic component that does not last very long. The fistula, on the other hand, is more naturally installed using our own body parts insuring the integrity of the installation, and the durability of its function.

Memoir
A More Humane Dialysis Center
07/04/01

My friend, Crystal, had quite an experience when she traveled last summer back east on vacation. I spoke with her prior to her leaving, and she was so excited about the trip. This would have been her first trip out of town since she became a renal patient. She was on her way to visit several cities and a couple of states on the east cost.

I missed Crystal's smile and her cheerful positive expression for the next two weeks. When I finally saw her again, I was happy to see her and asked her about her family and the trip in general. Crystal's glowing expression immediately transformed as she began to relate her experience. "The trip was alright. I was happy to see my mother and the rest of the family. What I wasn't ready for was the treatment I received from a dialysis center in N.J. They treated me like dirt. It was like I was doing them a big favor. I asked them for some pain killer before they stuck me with those big needles, and they just outright denied me. They treated me like they were doing me a big favor. They don't make you feel very welcome, and I'll tell you what, they don't have to worry about me going back there anymore."

"Crystal, I am so sorry that you had that kind of experience, but it makes me glad to see you back." I said, to encourage her. Crystal is truly an inspiration to most people. She is industrious. Besides going to her dialysis and working full time, she is pursuing a Bachelor's degree at a local university.

Crystal's experience is not an isolated case. I have heard this before. My concern here is that at times patients may feel that they have no support in the centers where they dialyze. I have heard the conversations of technicians reflecting such lack of care and professionalism. It really stems from poorly defined mission statements, goals, a lack of leadership and organizational training. A poorly managed center, in the area of staffing, training and development can easily attribute to ill prepared technicians. The mission of a center should be concerned with the patients well being. A sterile environment should be at the forefront of consideration.

I have experienced an environment where a number of patients have suffered from some staff infections due to inadequate procedures. I have learned that patients should reject such things as communal hot water bottles. Instead they should opt for a hot glove. The communal hot water bottle gets reused by different patients, and cross contamination and infection is eminent.

Dialysis centers must be prepared to provide the best care for their patient, not only because this should be their ultimate goal, but because as a business, they must be professionals as well.

In this business their customers or clientele can be young or old. They can range from the most knowledgeable patient, who follow every detail of their treatment, to those who are content to just flop in the chair and go along for the ride.

It behooves the centers administrators to adopt policies that keep their technicians and other professionals trained with the latest techniques and equipment to avoid embarrassing moments. It is one thing to have a new employee who is just too new to have mastered all the techniques. It is quite another, however, when you have employees who follow practices that are counterproductive to maintaining a sterile environment, as an example.

Memoir
A Therapeutic Journey
08/10/01

I have a birthday coming up in a couple of days. What I really want more than anything, right now, is to be able to travel. This disease has made it a very difficult thing to do these days but as you might have noticed by now, I do have a way of getting away through the memory of my experiences.

Have you ever had the spontaneous opportunity of just rising early in the morning and gotten in your car and just decided to drive? I did just that one early autumn day and headed west from the City of Denver on Interstate Seventy towards a mountain town by the name of Defiance, Colorado.

Have you ever heard of Defiance Colorado? Well, if you were ever an avid television buff during the mid-sixties when T.V. shows featured series of the untamed wild, wild west, you may have heard of Defiance. Defiance was the home town of the legendary western icon Doc Holiday.

Today the town is better known as Glenwood Springs. It is famous for its naturally heated mineral spring water (Hot Springs). Producing over four million gallons of water daily, tourist and visitors alike are attracted to it. Our history books teach that even before the white man discovered the springs in 1882, the Ute Indians had already been seen using the mineral water for medicinal purposes, and thus, the name "Yampah Hot Springs."

Nestled high in the Colorado Rockies between Vail and Aspen, it is only a few hours from Denver. This is an Ideal pit stop for travelers using Interstate Seventy in either direction.

First time travelers through this area will experience the awesome beauty of God's wondrous   creation, while viewing the collage of different colored mountains. Your automobile will be challenged by the steep incline of semi-arid hills and then meander into greener valleys of cedar and pine. You will crest the summit of the snow covered mountain tops and for a blissful moment become one with the clouds. In the rear view mirror of your car, you get the last peek of a winter wonder land being left behind. The blanket of white that once covered the mountain has been absorbed into the ground, revealing the red clay dirt that rushes down the mountain side to greet you. Your car dips and takes a couple of turns one to the left and then a right and with the power and sensation of a water slide, your car is flushed along side the infamous rushing white water of the Colorado River.

Skillful kayakers can be seen engaging the challenge of the white water on your left, while vertical slabs of solid rock canyon walls stretch their fingers to the sky.

Without seeming interested, you soak up the view like a sponge, as you negotiate the twists and turns of the canyons. Such exhilaration through the turn just brings out the child in you. It is reminiscent of the old Cyclone Roller Coaster in Brooklyn's Coney Island by the bay. Every youngster should have such a memory of an amusement park scene with cotton candy, Nathan's hot dogs and frog legs. Within a few minutes, you are out of the canyon and are now greeted by an almost conspicuous red sign in the side of the mountain that reads, "Yampah Hot Springs."

You are now in Glenwood Springs and your therapeutic trip has only just begun.

Memoir
Waking The Sleeping Giant
9/11/01

I have thought long and hard about the entries for this day. Well, I didn't have to go to dialysis today, like the world really cares! The world is busy today being in shocked. Yes, the shock of disbelief that the United States is under attack. The World Trade Center in New York City was attacked this morning.

After greeting the guard who stood at the main entrance to the building where I work, I was drawn to the monitor mounted high on the wall behind the guard's desk. The monitor displayed what appeared to be scenes from the movie "Towering Inferno". Why are they showing this movie at this time of the morning? It was rather inappropriate, I thought.   Normally, the weather or stock market reports are displayed. I didn't give much thought as I boarded the elevator for the third floor.

The workplace was in a panic. Some people listened to radios, while others, surfed the internet looking for news about New York City and the World Trade Center. Most workstations were locked in on CNN where spectacular pictures of a commercial plane seen colliding with one of the twin towers of the World Trade Center in lower Manhattan.

I had not been at work a good fifteen minutes before my wife called asking, if I had heard the news. She had been trying to call home to New York, but unable to get through to either my mother or hers. The phone lines were overloaded with calls.

On Monday, September 10th, the media's main attraction was Representative Gary Candid and aide, Chandra Levy. I was obsessed with a broken down, ill functioning kidney. People where preoccupied with their daily tasks. They operated out of their comfort zone; with their complaisant behavior, and today we all seek God's guidance and protection. The combined action of some twisted minds has turned our world inside out. It shocked us into reassessing our priorities.

It does not take much to upset the frail fabric of our society; whether it is the loss of a kidney or the bombing of our buildings, the destruction of a city or our ideals, our vulnerability becomes exposed. As a result, we now grieve our dead. We miss our former way of life, but most of all we are in shock that someone had the audacity to attack this great nation of ours. We are embarrassed, because no country is assuming the responsibility of the attack.

As a nation, we were hurt. As a people, we were devastated. The unthinkable has occurred. We thought that our once bought and paid for peace was to last forever, but those of a different mind set on September 11 proved to us that it was not forever.

The lesson here has been expensive and complicated as well. It has cost the lives of many people, billions of dollars in property damage, but most importantly we were awakened to the idea that there are those who not only do not embrace our idea of freedom and would go to their graves in an attempt to destroy it, and everything represented by it. Those people who have terrorized our country with such cowardly act of aggression have been labeled terrorists. For the longest, we have not taken them seriously. They have not only disrupted our lives, but, they have changed our way of living, and they most certainly have our attention now. Now that they have our attention are they happy. Are they satisfied or content or is their ends also their means, which is to continue in the path of destruction?

To have inflicted such an attack on the country and people of United States of America probably makes them feel a great sense of accomplishment. They probably feel like a worthy adversary. They might in fact have woken up a sleeping giant who is as faithful to its ideal of freedom as they are ready to die for their belief in destruction.

Memoir
Third Rail Adventure
10/17/01

Please forgive my digression from the subject of dialysis and renal malfunction. By now I am sure that you have realized that this book is not about dialysis and kidney failure, but rather about coping strategies that help us overcome the challenges in our lives. I realize that there is just so much more to life than our isolated individual misfortune. I must tell you that I am aware that there is nothing inspiring about enduring four hours of treatment in these clinics. In fact, it can be the most depressing environment if you are not able to get a hold of your mind.

I am thankful to God for allowing me the positive memories that I can retrieve and help me to cope. "Tio" is Spanish for Uncle. Tio has been a faithful depositor of positive memories in my life for some time now.

Tio's wife's name is Sylvia. Together they have two lovely daughters, Celina and Cecilia. As faith would have it, his youngest daughter Cecilia is also challenged by ESRD, (End Stage Renal Decease). One would hardly know this, since it has not deterred her purpose in life.

My cousin Cecilia is my heroin. After she was challenged with ESRD and complications regarding access for treatment, she pressed on with even a more focused mind to travel to Africa and complete ministry work. Since that time, Cecilia has gone on to complete her seminary program, and is now an ordained minister of the gospel of Jesus Christ. My Tio is proud of his daughter's accomplishments in the face of insurmountable odds, and I am too.

I want to share one of my Tio's adventures with you. Every time I hear the story of Tio's first visit to New York City it just cracks me up.

It must have been the middle of winter. The weather in the Big Apple was probably windy like Chicago's and just as cloudy and dreary looking as London, England. Tio had just arrived from the old country.

I think that you would like my Uncle George. He is tall, popular and just a likable kind of a guy. Because of his size, I believe he had very few takers. Those who know him would tell you that he is a giver. He is a big teddy bear. I always thought that the fox that scuffled with Tio inside grandma's chicken coop and left his signature under Tio's left eye could not have lived long, but that's a story for another time. To this day, he carries a scar prominently displayed on his left cheek serving as a reminder of an encounter with the fox that tried to steal grandma's chickens. That was in the old country, and I don't believe that the fox is still alive.

Compared to me Tio was a giant. Any one who knows me can confirm that I am closer to little people stature. I had nothing to fit Tio, but he was a survivor and protection from the elements was his only concern. The sleeves of the gray sweater he retrieved from the closet stretched itself at my uncle's forearm. The zipper did all it could but was unable to meet in the middle of his broad chest. Tio was happy to be in the United States with the rest of his small family. That is what made him happy, and if he could find some clothes that would fit him, well that would have been icing on the cake.

Tio explained the adventures of his experience while out looking for work. The enthusiasm in his voice as he described the different industrial neighborhood was very entertaining, to say the least. It was not because he was describing New York City, even though New York is deserving in itself. It is simply Uncle George's zeal for living and the things he encounters in his life. He has a way of making the most common and mundane appear as brand spanking new. He continued relating how he went here and there leaving work applications. His excursion led him to get off the subways at Green Way Plaza in Brooklyn. After taking care of his business, he stopped at a street cart vendor to get a quick lunch on the go. After inhaling the legendary New York hot dog, he boarded the subway homeward bound.

The names on the subway stop were unfamiliar to Tio. "No wonder I couldn't recognize any of these names. We are going in the wrong direction". He noted and immediately got off the train at the next stop. It dawned on him that he had spent the last of his money when he paid the vendor for the hot dog and orange soda he bought. Tio did not panic when he realized that he couldn't pay for another car fare. Without hesitation, he jumped down from the platform into the well of train tracks and proceeded to hop scotch across the tracks to the platform of the oncoming trains.

I asked Tio what was it like ? to run across the tracks with trains coming and going some not even stopping (the express trains). He said that he did not even think about it; but if he knew then what he knows know, that it wouldn't have crossed his mind to attempt such a foolish thing.

Anyone familiar with the Big Apple and its transportation system would agree that such an attempt would not be the wisest option for one to make. First of all, any hour of the day is considered rush hour in the city of New York. This may be a doable proposition at, night but certainly not at anytime during the day. I explained to Tio that he was placing himself in harms way, attempting to cross over six sets of tracks. The middle set is known as the express tracks, only stopping at certain designated stations. Each set of tracks is accompanied by a single third rail. That makes four additional tracks. This third rail is somewhat shielded, since it is the electrical source that powers the trains.

I always thought that my uncle was one of the bravest men I ever knew. I have admired the way that he traveled throughout the countries in Latin America. He is challenged by the unknown, not only the set of tracks where the train will be visibly traveling down, but there is the invisible voltage of the third rail that is always present. His execution must be perfectly timed to avoid the trains on eight tracks and at the same time, avoid the third rail voltage on four tracks. At the time, my uncle did not realize that the third rail carried enough punch to zap his lights out for good.

I was fascinated with the passion that he has for living. Almost everything that he does, is accomplished with intensity and much vigor. I can almost visualize his intense expression as he challenged the course across the train tracks.

I don't know when my uncle found out that this particular adventure was really unnecessary. The fact of the matter is that all he needed to do was to use the stairs up and over to the other side. This would have put him on the other side of the tracks, and it also would have been the most economical and safest alternative for travel in the opposite direction.

Memoir
Ground Zero
02/17/02

While surfing the web, I was surprised to find that there was a dialysis center right in my mother's neighborhood in Queens, New York. I called the center on Guy Brewer Boulevard and arranged to have my blood service right there in Queens while I visited my mother. After hearing of Crystal's experience in New Jersey, I must tell you that it made me a bit nervous not knowing whether the manifestation of a similar fate awaited me.

As much as New York City has to offer, the casual visitor if their dialysis experience turns out to be a bad one, then there goes the rest of the trip. Fortunately, for me, it went well. Thank God for the standardization of the dialysis procedure. It seems that there is a network of facilities throughout the nation and maybe even throughout the world. I have been to three facilities in the United States and found them to be synchronized as far as information, procedures, and techniques are concerned. The advent of technology such as the fax machine makes communication within the network possible, especially the instantaneous transmission of one's medical records otherwise known as a run sheet for the purpose of dialyzing. I observed a major difference in the procedure between the Queens, New York Center, and the Denver, Colorado Center, even though they both belong to the same Davita organization. Patients who had a perm catheter installed in their chest, as I had, could not be put on or taken, (start or terminate their run) off their run by technical staff people. Only professional nurses are qualified to perform these procedures. Nurse Eunice Kwami further explained that it is not because they are not capable. Since the work is to be performed within a close proximity to the heart, at a major artery, the skills and responsiveness of a nurse is preferred. In fact, I believe that she said, it was the law in the state of New York.

My best friend John, who now lives in New Jersey came to Queens and was a personal guide for my mother, my wife and myself on a trip to Manhattan to visit the site of Ground Zero.

We took the Jackie Robinson freeway from Queens into Brooklyn. I believe Johnny wanted to show us the old neighborhood on Chauncey Street in Brooklyn.

1784 Broadway is what the address read as I looked up at the numbers. The "L" (short for elevated train) ran right by my windows, roaring like a pride of lions flexing the tracks beneath the weight of screeching wheels with tons of steel and the strength of a thousand horses. I can still hear the intervals of roaring crescendo as the train approached from several blocks away, reminding me of when mom and dad first moved to that address. When we first moved there I used to stay awaked nights wondering how in the world I would ever get accustomed to this noise. It wasn't long before the noise of the train was assimilated into our daily habits and hardly noticeable any longer.

We continued the scenic route underneath the L, up Broadway past Halsey Avenue, and then finally took a right turn on to Gates Avenue, where John lived.

Let me tell you about Halsey Avenue. This was a train stop midway between Gates Ave. where John lived and Chauncey Ave where I lived. We normally spent the evenings on John's stoop, playing stick ball in the street or just sitting around telling jokes and talking about girls. When it was time to go home, that was around 8:30 p.m., John was supposed to walk me half way, but we were so engrossed in our conversation, that by the time we realized it he had walked me all the way home. We did the next best thing just stood at my stoop and talked some more. John would then mention that he walked me all the way home, insinuating that maybe this wasn't just. I would then turn around and walk him back. Finally, he walked me back half way, which was Halsey Street. We couldn't figure out why couldn't we have thought of this before now.

Yeah, there is the stoop where we hung out in the evenings after dinner and home work was done. We played stick ball in the middle of the street, until it got dark and then just sat there on the stoop talking about girls or playing horse until it was time to go in.

"Charles you remember the gas station that used to be right there on the corner by my house"? John asked me. I should tell you now that we called each other Charles since junior high school. "Yeah, I remember the station."

I replied, "But there is something different! there doesn't seem to be anything new or even missing so why did they take the station away". It looked like the place I knew, but there was something different I just couldn't put my finger on it. "What they did, interrupted John, " was, build two more three family houses right next to mine. Can you see it now?" John was right. The two additional residential buildings right next to his, blended without changing the neighborhood.

It was a very sunny day, a bit chilly, but otherwise nice. Charles continues to cruise the scenic route until we got downtown Brooklyn. He wanted to show us the new Brooklyn sea shore. Charles said that the old Fulton Street Fish Market had been moved and replaced with the new Brooklyn Sea Shores. For some reason, we didn't get to see either, but before we knew it, we were at the entrance of the Brooklyn Bridge.

Greeting us as we got onto the bridge where a couple of New York's finest armed with what appeared to be semi-automatic riffles, and a sad melancholic expression that seem to carry the burden of the entire city of New York. After the bridge, it was a turn here and a turn there, and before you knew it, we were there; a big pit in the ground, better known as Ground Zero.

Why we call this place ground zero? I'll never know. You see, ground zero was used to describe the location of a nuclear bomb explosion; nonetheless, we were there.

133

We walked around where John suggested and took some pictures while he explained what took place on that infamous date of September 11. I was glad that my mother was able to get out of the house with us and get a breath of fresh air. My friend retold the once in a lifetime horrifying experience that he wished New Yorkers never had to go through. Most of the graphic descriptions are best left untold, but there is one that I wish to share with you.

John worked in a building directly across from the World Trade Center in lower Manhattan. He lives in Piscataway, New Jersey about an hour's commute to get to work by train. A typical morning for Charles would be to drive his car to the train station. He would have breakfast and mingle with passengers at a neighborhood restaurant before boarding the train at approximately the same time everyday. John would ride the train with the same people at the same time, and get off at the World Trade Center stop.

The event of 911 has changed people in just about every walk of life. It didn't matter how far away, or how close you might have been to the occurrence. For people who must still commute to lower Manhattan from Piscataway, well, they must find a different way to get there. That train stop is no longer there. John's employer relocated him temporarily somewhere in New Jersey. Since John no longer commutes to Manhattan, he can drive to his new location, instead of to the train station to mingle and have breakfast.

Several months have passed since John visited the little neighborhood restaurant by the train station. So he thought that he would drop by and pay everyone there a surprise visit. Was he ever surprised at what he found! The proprietor looked at him with great astonishment. After pausing for a brief moment, he then ran over to John and grabbed him by his shoulder's and began feeling his arms like he was checking some produce in the super market for firmness. "Is it really you Johnny? My God you are alive. Hey Guz it's Johnny! He's alive. We all thought that you were dead, Johnny. I am going to tell the others that you are alive." Johnny did not know what to reply, so he just said, "Yeah, please tell them that I am alive."

It just didn't occur to John that he should have returned to the restaurant soon after the 911 events to let them know that he was not a casualty. "What's even worse, Johnny" is the apparent abandonment of all those vehicles that have been parked at the train station ever since 911. Will their owners ever be back to claim them?"

Memoir
Lovie's Story

Jorge Joseph Taylor

I remember it like it was yesterday. It was late August towards the end of my tour in Saint Petersburg. I was sitting in my office in Saint Petersburg when my manager broke the news to me about an assignment in New York City. I could barely contain the excitement inside of me. I have always loved NYC, and thought I would like to live there some day, right in the middle of Manhattan. It had been several years since I last visited NYC, so I was thinking of all of the things I would do when I was not working; Broadway shows, visiting Harlem, shopping, shopping, riding the ferry, etc. This assignment was to last through at least March of 2002. Six months in NYC!!! Then my manager indicated that I would love the view from the office. What view could this be I wondered? All I could imagine was building after building, so any view from an office would probably be looking at another building. Then my manager said, "your office will be on the 97th floor of the World Trade Center". I can still vividly recall how my legs began to shake from my fear of the height. Yes, I was petrified of height. However, I could not bring myself to let my manager know this. I said to myself, "you will sound like and be viewed as a wimp", so just plan to go into the office every day and do not look down.

So on Sept 10, I traveled from Boulder to NYC. My trip started with a Super Shuttle ride from Boulder to the Denver airport. When I arrived at the airport, I discovered that my watch was missing. After tracing my steps, I was convinced that I had lost it, or maybe I would recover it after returning home in a few weeks. Even to this day, I have not found it nor do I understand why I was not to have a watch on the day of Sept 11.

My flight from Denver to LaGuardia International Air Port was a smooth one. I spent most of the flight re-reading chapters from a book that I had bought earlier that summer in Florida. It was an exposition on Positive Thinking, by Dr. Vincent Peale. Upon arriving at La Guardia Air Port, I began to experience an involuntary transition to another level. I automatically stored away Dr. Peale's observation on positive thinking. In fact, this new venue was completely opposite. There was no time left for the art of any kind of thinking. My adrenalin began pumping, and suddenly I was there. It wasn't gradually, like cars blending into traffic by means of merging lanes, no, not like that. It was more like the Star Ship Enterprise bound by the earthly gravitational laws in one instance, and then whala! Warp speed, and you are there.

I began to feel an irregular pulse in the air, even before we touched down. It seemed like every one had been drinking from the same water and contacted the same epidemic. Then again that couldn't be true either, because I have not had a drink. Yet I feel as much affected by this frenzy as every one else. It must be something in the air and not in the water. No, a sort and frenzy epidemic that no one seems able to escape. It is the diversity of the Big

Apple. It is truly different. The coined phrase "in a New York minute" really came alive for me. I felt like I was playing a leading role in a James Bond feature film.

I took a cab to the Marriott Hotel that was across the street from the World Trade Center (W.T.C.) in lower Manhattan. This is actually the beginning tip of Manhattan. After I checked in and received a room on the 38th floor, I began to re-live my fear of heights. I really wanted to ask for a lower floor, but decided otherwise, thinking that I might as well start getting used to the height if I was to be in New York City for any length of time.

I entered the room slowly. After placing my bags down, I continued gradually towards the window to see how I would feel. I noticed that it had begun to rain. The fog was setting in over the Hudson. As I got to the window, I felt a bit queasy, but I was able to look out the window onto the river and calm the unrest, if only momentarily, about my fear of heights.

The first thing that I would do when I reached my hotel was to call home, communicate with my husband, Coy and call my daughter, Carolyn, in Evanston, Illinois.

My husband, Coy, shared my excitement of being in NYC. When he answered the phone, he wanted to know how it felt to be in the Big Apple. Unlike my husband, my daughter Carolyn did not appear to share in my excitement.

When I called her, she showed no excitement. In fact, I can recall the sick feeling that I got from her lack of reaction on the phone. I did not say anything to her, but I wondered why she was acting so emotionless. This was so out of character for her. In the past, she was always excited when I shared my travel experiences of places that I had never been to. She would ask me about how I planned to spend my time when not at work. She knew that I loved being adventurous and exploring new cities and neighborhoods for their cultural activities. This excitement was just not there with her on that day. As I reflect now, I think that God was preparing me for something to come.

My evening was spent in the hotel with dinner in my room. I had gone downstairs to go out to eat, but it was raining so hard, I decided to stay in. On Tuesday morning, I woke up, prayed for a while then read a chapter from Psalms, cannot recall the chapter. I was anxious to get to the office as early as possible but realized that this was NYC, and the work day did not start as early as in Denver. Also I wanted to get there so I could meet everyone. I had not met any of the people who worked for my company nor the customer.

So, I decided that I would get there by 8 am. I went down the hall to the concierge's room to have some breakfast. I was not hungry, but forced myself to eat some fruit. I took a bottle of water and returned to my room. I gathered my laptop carrying case, put my bottle in it, and headed for the office.

As I began to open the door, a strong feeling hit me, I stopped closed the door and stood there and started praying again. I said, "God, I know that through You all things are possible". Now, I was so focused on doing a good job on this assignment, I was praying for great customer satisfaction. Little did I know what He, (God) had in store to show me what He can make possible. Afterward, I went downstairs and across the street to the World Trade Center WTC/Tower 2. It was probably about five minutes before 8 a.m. I had been told to go to the information booth on the first floor to get my photo ID done so that I could come in and out of the building everyday. The lobby area was buzzing with people.

My NYC excitement began to grow more and more; I was looking forward to the crowds of people, taxi cabs, sirens, etc of the Big Apple. I found the information booth and was surprised that it only took a few minutes to get the photo ID done. Then I was told to, use it to get thru the turnstile to get to one of the elevators. The time is now about 8:10a.m. Well, my "country bumpkin, slow-pace Denver mindset" kicked in. Which turnstile? There were quite a few, tried one, could not figure it out quickly, felt uncomfortable, because I did not want to hold up any line for these fast moving New Yorkers. So, I moved down to the last one to my left and asked the security person for help. Actually, this New Yorker was nice and gladly helped me. Got on the elevator, took it to the 78th floor, and then had to transfer to another elevator to get to the 97th floor.

On the first elevator, I saw this familiar man, and tried to figure out if I had seen him on the plane the day before or in the hotel. When we got off the elevator on the 78th floor, he got on the next elevator before I did. I continued to try to figure out why he looked so familiar. As the elevator door closed, he called my name, and then right away it came back to me where I had seen him. I had met him in California the previous Friday. He was my customer that I had only met once for a brief moment. He was so warm and excited that I would come and take on this challenge to work through the customer satisfaction issues. He said that he was looking forward to meeting with me and another person that afternoon. He thought the meeting would be around 1 p.m. but maybe a little later. I told him that I appreciated the opportunity and not to worry about the time because I would be there for some months. I was not going anywhere. He got off, I think, on the 93rd floor.

When I reached the 97th floor, I discovered that I still needed someone to get me into the office. Fortunately, someone was coming out, and I asked if they could get me to my contact. Upon entering the office area of the 97th floor, all I could see were windows, windows, windows; no outer solid walls, all outer walls are windows. The fear was in control again. I told myself to look straight ahead, do not look down. My contact's work area was on the outer aisle next to the window. I met my contact, talked a few minutes with him, then he started taking me around to meet members of my company's team and some of the customers. As we were leaving his work area, I told myself to try to look down to see how it would feel. I did and ABSOLUTELY no shaking of the knees or sweaty palms. Wow, I said to myself, this is a piece of cake; I got it, won't be a problem for me. Little did I know what He was preparing me for? How quickly I starting thinking that I was the one that had removed this fear. The time I would think would probably be between 8:15 and 8:20a.m. We continued on for the next 20 to 25 minutes meeting people. We approached the desk of a colleague who immediately stood up, and I was introduced to Lenny. Yes, Lenny. I could only smile and nod as Lenny began to speak, because I could not understand most of what he was saying. He had a very strong, strong Eastern European accent.

Lenny extended a bag of wrapped candy out to me. Initially, my thoughts were to say "No" because I thought to myself, "I don't want any candy this early in the morning nor do I need any". Then something within me said," He is reaching out to you, take the candy. A small piece of candy is not going to make your already excess pounds any worse." I took a piece, intending still to just put it in my pocket for later. Then he offered a piece to

Mark, fortunately Mark's reply of "no" was gruff and sharp. Within I said, "Lovie!, eat the candy in front of Lenny to let him know that you appreciate it". I removed the candy's wrapper and started to eat it. Then thanked Lenny and told him I would see him later. Little did I know that it would be sooner rather that later?

Mark and I headed back to his work area. However, we were stopped by one of our customers. The person asked Mark if he was going to the 9am DR (disaster recovery) meeting. Since I had lost my watch, I had to look at Mark's watch to see what time it was. It was exactly 8:45a.m. Mark indicated "yes" but needed a few minutes to get access cards for me so that I could get in and out of the office area on that floor. So we continued on back to his work area. I stopped next to Mark's work area, because I saw a colleague that I had worked with in Florida. We began to chat. At that point, I am standing facing east. I heard a loud noise, similar to a sonic boom, looked to my left (north) and saw this HUGE BALL of fire. I could tell that it was outside of the building that I was in. It looked like it was between the 2 buildings. The ball of fire quickly became a HUGE BALL of smoke; the flame disappeared like it had come from a blow torch. When the sound of the explosion was first heard, someone/a man's voice yelled out, "Oh my God. There has been an explosion", and then seconds later, "Oh my God, it is in building one". People began to stand up from their work areas in shock. Some

145

moved toward the north windows to see what was going on. From out of the crowd a voice cried out, "Oh My God, a plane has hit the building". I remember standing where I was and seeing a very tall customer who I had met earlier stand up. He began to wave his hands, indicating the folks should move to the south end of the building. Many of us followed him to the south end. It was pretty much a "white out" on the outside from the south windows. There was so much paper, bits of paper floating around in the air, and I guess some of it was smoke. We started going to the south end of the building. I am thinking that we are going to take the stairs or something. Instead, I recall that this very tall customer and another woman attempted to make contact with someone via phone. However, they discovered that the phones were dead. This very tall customer indicated that we should go back to the other end. As I returned to the place that I was originally standing, Lenny was there saying "Lovie, come on let's go". Now, I understand clearly every word that Lenny was saying. Thank God!! I grabbed my purse and computer bag. Also, I said to Mark (from San Fran), "come on let's go." Mark was taking his time, wrapping neatly his computer power supply cord. Lenny again said, "Lovie, come on, let's go"! At that point, I felt that I should go with Lenny, so I quickly started to follow him. We headed for the stairs, by this time Mark had caught us with us. The stairs were full with people, moving quickly, but no panic that I could see or hear. My purse and computer bag became heavy and cumbersome to carry as we moved down the stairs. So, as I was trying to adjust them to ease the weight, Lenny took the computer bag and said he would carry it. Then it hit me that maybe I needed to shed that computer bag and leave it there. Lenny insisted that he could carry it.

An announcement from the building's PA system started somewhere around when we were on the 80-ish floor (don't remember exact floor). The announcement indicated that "the fire is in Building One, Building Two is safe, go back to your work area". It was repeated over and over and over. Lenny said "Keep going". I think that many people were thinking like I was that a plane had hit the building by accident due to pilot error. I had visualized a small plane. However, when we reached the 78th floor, Lenny and others left the stairwell and went to the elevators. The 78th floor was the transfer floor for the elevators. In the meantime, the announcement is still going about returning to your work area. As we approach the elevators, I am trying to retrieve my cell phone, from my purse, so that I can call Coy to let him know what is going on with me. I knew he would be watching CNN news and probably hear/see that a plane had hit one of the WTC buildings. He did not know which building I was in. I was unsuccessful in getting a dial tone, in the meantime, just as we got to the elevators, one opened up right in front of me. It was completely empty. Lenny is saying "Get on". As I am getting on, and with the announcement still repeating, I look over to the bank of elevators that go from 78 up, I see John enter one to go back up. I wanted to yell out and say "no John, do not go back up"!

The elevator from the 78th floor went straight to the 1st floor within seconds, no stops. The elevator was pretty full, but not packed tightly. When we got to the 1st floor, I thought we would exit the building by going to the left and entering the street. The many, many police officers and firemen in the lobby directed us to the right and thru the revolving doors to the passageway that commuters took to the subway on a daily basis. I understand that this was the underground mall, because we passed all types of shops as we were walking. This area was packed with people, moving hurriedly, not to much panic. Police officers and firemen were also in this passageway in great numbers, asking people to move quickly, and stay calm.

Then, there were two booming sounds, sounds of explosions, loud but not shaking. I thought that these were sounds of more explosions from the fire in Building One, caused the plane hitting the building. However, after hearing folks screaming "oh my God, they have hit this building", I knew that something bad was going on. Mark (from San Fran) grabbed and hugged me, crying. The police officers raised the tone in their orders and said, "people, get out of here quickly, move fast, move, move, don't panic, but move, move!," We arrived at an intersection in the mall passageway; we could have gone straight ahead or made a left. Lenny said, "This way". We made a left. I did not see which direction Mark took. As I turned left, I could see sunlight. There was a flight of escalator steps that would take you up to street level. Many people were waiting in line to take the side of the escalator going up. But Lenny went over to the one going down and said, " Lovie, over here". I thought to myself, "This will be hard to try to go up escalator steps that are coming down". However, I remember stepping on the first step and stepping off at the top, no struggle, no pain. Again the police officers were ordering people to move quickly and get away from the building. People were actually stopping and looking up to try to see what was happening. Lenny told me to keeping going which I did. We headed east, moving hurriedly. The crowds of people were pretty much on the sidewalks, because rescue trucks and cars were using all lanes of the street, headed to the buildings.

The sidewalks were packed with people, crying, screaming, in panic as we continued to walk, I could hear people talking about other planes were still in the air. I am trying desperately to get through to Coy and Carolyn on my cell phone. No success. But we continue to walk. I don't recall how far away from the building we were or what time it was, but I heard in the back of me these screams that the building was coming down. Now people took over the streets, running away from the buildings. Lenny told me at that time, "Lovie, keep going, don't look back, keep going!" I did not look back. So I never saw the crumbling of the buildings as others did or those who watched it on TV. We continued to walk. Lenny wanted to know if I were going home to Colorado. I told him that I could not because people were saying that all airports were closed. He was worried about me being away from my family.

As we walked Lenny kept asking if I was able to get through to my family on my cell phone. I wanted to stop to try to use a public phone, but Lenny would not let me. He said "Lines too long, we keep walking". I was also concerned about him making contact with his family. I learned that he lived in New Jersey and that his family should be ok. His wife worked in Manhattan, but probably had not left home because of her start time for work. So we continued to walk. I was receiving many, many messages on my pager from colleagues and friends, but could not respond, because cell phones were not working. Finally, after walking for blocks and blocks, Lenny indicated that we should try to use a public phone where the line was fairly short. I tried to call home, but the call kept going to voice mail. I think, that by this time so many folks were calling Coy, trying to find out if he had heard from me. Next, I called Carolyn's office in Evanston. Her co-worker answered and told me that Carolyn had left the office to go back home. Rather than make another call and not let the next person in line try to contact their loved ones, I asked

Carolyn's co-worker to call Carolyn, have Carolyn call her father, the rest of the family and my manager. Then I made a call for Lenny, and he spoke to someone to get the word to his family that he was safe.

Then we continued to walk. I thanked Lenny so many times. I told him to try to get home, and I would be ok. However, I had no idea what I would do. He insisted that he would stay with me and we would continue to walk. I guess to New Jersey. We stopped around 1 p.m. to get water and have something to eat. I ordered a sandwich along with Lenny, but was not hungry, could not even think of food. Lenny and I ate one of the 2 sandwiches. Then we continued to walk.

About 2 p.m. I insisted that we stop and try to call his family again so he could speak directly to them. The connection to New Jersey did not work. I called a colleague in Florida, who connected Lenny to his family. Also, they connected us to our company's crisis line, where we were told where to go for refuge. I certainly did not know where we were or where this company's location was. But, I asked Lenny and he said, "I know. I know". So we continued to walk, arriving at our company uptown location about 4: 30p.m.

Our company crisis team was there in FULL FORCE to take care of us. The medical staff checked us out, made sure that we made contact with family, had food, etc. Guess who was already at the location?, Mark, from

San Fran. He has been with the company for many years and knew about this location. Also, two other colleagues from out of town had made their way to the location. The crisis team tried to find hotels for us that night, but was not successful. We spent the night at the office; the crisis team made makeshift beds with cushions from sofas from various offices and tablecloths from the cafeteria as the sheets.

On Wednesday, Lenny was sent home to New Jersey by car service. Hotel rooms were found for the rest of us. Also, we were sent out shopping for clothes, since none of us could get back to our hotels. We received more medical attention on Wednesday afternoon and the beginning of crisis counseling. Airports were still all shut down so we knew that we could not get back to our homes. I was in constant communications with family, friends and colleagues, praying and rejoicing about the miracle with me. I had a conversation with my manager on

Wednesday night and indicated that since I could not get home to Colorado, I wanted to try to get to New Jersey to the site where we were helping our customer to get back in business. Arrangements were made for us to rent a car and to drive to New Jersey.

We arrived in New Jersey around midnight on Thursday and went directly to the work location. I stayed in New Jersey until Friday, September 21st. Working 18 to 20-hour days, every day.

I thank God for His Mercy and Grace that day!!! He truly was with me. There were so many miracles that day. I am told that the second plane was held on the runway for 18 minutes at the Boston-Logan airport. The plan was that both planes would hit at the same time. The second plane hit the second building/Tower 2 around the 80th floor. No one above that point had a chance. My office was on the 97th floor. Also, when I thought that I had conquered the fear of height all by myself earlier that day, I now know that God was preparing me for the events that were coming within the hour. As we walked down those stairs, NEVER did my heart race fearfully out of control. I knew that I needed to move quickly, but I was not afraid. I even recall when we were outside, and the word of more plane attacks and other threats of attacks, I said to myself, "Manhattan is an island, it could easily be blown up, I said this might be the day that I will see My Heavenly Father, I did not cry out in fear, I said to myself that I know that Carolyn will take care of her father and my brothers and sisters would know that I loved the Lord and had tried to serve Him" So I was at peace. I learned months later Lenny who had a friend that was at the door of the same elevator where I was. He beckoned her to get in, she nodded and said no that she would take the next one, I don't know if there was another elevator but she did not make it out.

Where did Lenny Belvasky come from why did I meet him? Why did he offer me candy? What happened to the customer that I saw going back towards the office. Did he ever make it out alive?   I have many unanswered questions, as a result of that one day. Twenty-four hours after the tragedy, I was contacted and asked to describe what he was wearing to the media. Any hope of finding him alive became dimmer over the course of the next two weeks.

In October many of his family members came to New York, and asked if I would consider meeting them. I met them one Saturday morning, and I spent the entire day with them.

I will forever be indebted to Lenny for his obedience to God. Lenny puts it this way: he thanks God for letting him help me Lenny and I keep in close touch today.

Memoir
Cardiovascular Research
02/28/02

The biggest snow storm of the season was predicted for this afternoon; the same time of Dr. Block's dinner presentation. Dr. Geoffrey Block is my Nephrologists. During his monthly visitation at the dialysis clinic, he shared with me that he has been conducting a research project involving heart decease. He said that in the past, most of his presentations were aimed at other professional doctors. Never before had he presented his findings, (in his own words) to "the people that it really affects, the patients themselves". He seemed very excited as he asked if we planned to attend.

The location of the event was The Presbyterian Saint Luke's Hospital in downtown Denver. The medium size theater style auditorium was packed.

I was surprised that I recognized most of the attendees. Most were dialysis patients and their families. My wife and I managed to find two seats close together in the front row. Before we could get comfortable, the young Dr. Block was addressing the gathering crowd. He encouraged us to make our way back to the buffet line, and maybe, if we were timely, we could get done with dinner and lecture before the menacing storm of the century arrives.

Dinner was ready.

The term gentleman and a scholar seemed to fit the young doctor well. What a guy! Knowing that, he was to be requiring our undivided attention during his presentation, he thought it best to feed us first. He catered in a buffet-style dinner with a choice of turkey, gravy or baked chicken.

The Dr. stood between two video projection screens as he spoke. The screens angled off in opposite directions towards the viewing audience.

Dr. Block began his presentation by telling us that what he was about reveal was frightening.

I can't say that I disagree with him. It's just that this is a sort of an understatement. What is frightening is realizing that, by the grace of God, we were given another chance at living. What's frightening is to realize that I was crossing over into another dimension when I got snatched from the jaws of death.

Dr. Block says that there is phosphorous in almost everything that we eat. The presence of vitamin D in the body allows the body to absorb phosphorous. The problem is that the ESRD patient's PTH, (Para Thyroids Hormones stops), producing the necessary vitamin D. This results in an irregular PTH value. A high PTH value drives the calcium out of the bone. The calcium seems to vanish from the body, because it cannot be found anywhere. This is not entirely true. The calcium deposits itself into the tissue of the heart.

This is what is frightening. The calcium never leaves the body. Calcium is good for calcifying strong teeth and bones, and maybe even a heart. Yes Dr. Block says that the calcium traces are ending up inside the tissue of the heart. The only weapon to combat the calcium and phosphorous problem is a controlled consumption of calcium, phosphorous and the use of food binder's such as Renagel or phoslo.

The business of phosphorous, calcium, and other chemical balance in our system is such a sensitive matter that this medicine environment seems more like an art than the science that people seem to ascribe to it. It is a concern that I would rather avoid if possible. I cannot wait for the opportunity of a new kidney. Until that happens, Dr. Block says "we need the right amount of calcium X phosphorous, (CaXP) product, to maintain a balance of healthy bones and teeth. A high Ca x P product(calcium X Phosphorus) can lead to calcium deposits in your joints, organs, and blood vessels. These calcium deposits are called "metastatic calcification". High phosphorus can cause weak bones."

Memoir
The Boy King
04/20/02

I must have been about nine years old when my grandma dressed us up to go to the parade. It was during the mid- nineteen fifties, and the city was cleaning up and prepping up for one of the biggest events of its kind to take place. It was the visit of the royal family of England. The Queen herself, Queen Elizabeth was to be parading down Main Street. My grand mother was most exited about the queen's visit. The motorcade came and went down the street with Her highness waving from side to side at the throng of people lined the street on either side.

Granny new much about England's Monarchy! I remember her complementing me about how well dressed I looked, comparing me to some duke or royal member of Buckingham palace.

It has taken about fifty years for me to see another King. Only this time it is African Royalty, and only a boy of (10) ten years of age. King Oyo Nyimba Kabamba Iguru Rukidi IV was crowned King of The Toros Kingdom in Uganda, Southern Africa at the age of three, making him the youngest reigning king on record.

I remember not feeling well on the Sunday evening of the Kings visit to our city. The ministerial alliance of the city of Denver had arranged for the king to have a reception at my church. All my kids had made their way down to the church but me.

It didn't take me long to realize that I had to get down to the church. I wanted to be apart of this most memorable occasion.

King Oyo has been an ambassador for his country. He travels around the world soliciting funds for the creation of a new hospital to help to combat the Aids epidemic. This disease has left Uganda with the highest orphan rate than any other country in the world. As I watched the young King Oyo preside from his throne, for that moment I was no longer aware of the discomfort that I suffered from the excess fluids accumulating in my body. I could not help but think that this young boy must be full of desire to be like others his age out playing, having fun, and just enjoying the fruits of their youth. The noble calling of this young king is to make a difference for all the other children in his kingdom. It was uplifting and encouraging to have witnessed the conviction, dedication, and sacrifice of this young ten-year old boy King. If this little boy could suck it up and roll up his sleeves and leave his childhood games behind him, in order to pursue the greater purpose for the subject of his kingdom, maybe there is hope for an old man like myself. Maybe I too can focus on the greater purpose ordained by Jesus himself when he commanded us in Matthew 28:19 to go forth into all the world teaching and preaching.

Memoir
Choosing Death
05/01/02

Two and a half years have now passed since I was first admitted to the hospital for this kidney disease. I have learned much since then. I have observed many physically limiting circumstances invade the human body; I have watched the crippling and imprisonment of the mind, and the oppression of evil spirits as they enslave and hold the human spirit hostage against its own will.

In an earlier chapter, I mentioned the options of treatments available against kidney decease. They are as follow: Hemodialysis, Peritoneal dialysis, kidney transplant, and of course, not making any of these choices would be a choice in itself. The resulting lack of action will inevitably lead to one's death.

For the first time, I have met someone who opted to abstain from making a life sustaining choice. To protect her identity let's call her Sarah.

Sarah was a very quiet person. She had not been at the center for very long. She had a small frame, a petite size woman who slipped away just as quietly as she had arrived at the center, with little or no commotion at all.

The evil cancer cells had increasingly gained control of the territory of Sarah's frail body. The chemotherapy treatment could not keep pace with the advances of this disease. It was a day late and a dollar short. Sarah was tired. The fight had left her body. One day she asked her renal doctor what kind of death she would suffer as a result of not continuing with dialysis. She knew that death would come in the end, but she wanted to know how much would she suffer. The doctor informed her that it would probably be a quiet death in her sleep.

Sarah opted to discontinue dialysis treatment and registered herself into one of the local hospice centers. Two weeks hadn't passed before she died. Life continues in Sarah's absence. Things continue to be better sometimes and worse at other times. Her children are no longer burdened with the challenge of having to bring her to dialysis and take her back home every other day. Maybe she will be missed tremendously by her family. One thing we know for sure is that she does not have to suffer the pain of those raving cancer cells in her body nor the cramping and tiresome feeling in her body every other day from the dialysis treatments.

I often wonder if Sarah was as concerned with the salvation of her soul as she was with pain in her body. I just wonder whether the question of eternity, salvation, and God crossed her mind at all. I neglected to tell her about Jesus' saving grace. I will probably have to answer for that. I only hope now that someone was concerned enough to tell her about Jesus Christ. Well what does it matter now? Sarah's opportunity is a thing of the past much like water under the bridge.

As far as we know, death is pretty final. Life is not a dress rehearsal. Contrary to what we may have heard or want to believe regarding reincarnation, God's word is clear when it states that it has been appointed once for man to die. The statement "life is not a dress rehearsal", means only one thing. We only have one shot at life. We do not get a second chance to get it right. It does not matter whether our chance ends with September 11th or whether it ends because we opted not to continue our dialysis treatment. Once we are out, we are out. It is not only impossible to undo what was done or make up whatever we had lacked doing for others, but time runs out regarding our own salvation too.

Choosing to die may be an option but how can we be so sure when death is so final. Choosing death is in deed the most critical choice one could make when considering the irreversible character of such a choice.

Memoir
I Know What My Will Is
05/05/02

Today I go back to the hospital for a procedure commonly referred to as a CT scan.

I am to have one of these procedures every year to determine if the cancer remains gone.

It is said that once you have survived this disease, the chance of a recurrence is greater than for those who never had the disease.

If after two years there are no signs of this cancer, then I am allowed to get an appointment with the transplant people. This would make my whole clan happy, and of course, it would make me happy to.

My kidney doctor would rather that I don't pursue the transplant route, but go the peritoneal dialysis way. He feels that two years is not enough time to minimize the risk of recurrence. I believe that he would prefer that I would opt to stay on dialysis for the rest of my life.

My wife understands my doctor's point of view. She has become comfortable with the challenges that dialysis presents. She is afraid of the uncharted waters of the transplant procedure and the added complications of cancer disease. With no disrespect towards the medical profession or to my wife, my biological clock is ticking and I want to return to a wholesome life before its last tick. This is my own perspective. It is what I want, and then there is God. It is not a far fetched idea that God would want me whole, and if that is His will there isn't any amount of medical science or theory that can with hold it from me.

I always felt that getting to the transplant table would be my greatest challenge.

During the initial stages of dialysis treatment, I asked the doctor what does it take for me to be whole again. He told me in no uncertain terms that I would be sick for the rest of my natural life. The closest thing to restoration would be a kidney transplant. That's it? A kidney transplant. Sounded like a very doable proposition to me, except that there was more.

A tumor was discovered on my left kidney. Analysis of the tumor will be necessary to determine if it is malignant or benign. The result would determine my eligibility for the transplant list.

The question now is, is it God's will that I be healed completely or is it His will that I persevere in my condition and serve him from there. This is in deed a dilemma. I don't know if it is possible to be objective in this dilemma. I don't know if that is possible, because my will gets in the way. I want to be completely healed. I know that God is able, but the real question is, does my wants fall into the scope of His will. His will may be to increase the number of laborers in this particular vineyard. Honestly, if this was your call, what would you say? Don't be afraid to tell the truth, even though it may be different from His will. He Himself has said that His will is not like ours. This dilemma bothered me so much that I had to seek consultation. I will tell you about that later.

I want to serve the Lord, but if I had the choice, I believe that I would request a different vineyard. Wait a minute, maybe it has nothing to do with the vineyard; maybe it's just my personal circumstances. Yes, that's exactly what it is. I just want to be healed. Sometimes I feel that I have learned what it takes to cope with this environment, but then I begin to have dreams that ignore the barriers of my circumstances. My mind just takes flight and entertains visions that take me away from my circumstances.

As a kid I was a notorious dreamer. I would get away in a minute. I don't know if you were like me. If I was lucky enough to get a seat near a window in any class room, all I needed was a glimpse of a tree, or some clouds of cotton outside the window, and I was gone. I believe it was called day dreaming.

This very moment, as I dialyze in this center, the trees outside my window are getting bombarded with hail, and their leaves are being swept away by a strong gust of wind, and my memory flashes back to the days of the marching band.

Memoir
Marching Band
05/20/02

The cloud burst was sudden and without a warning. From the protective covering of my favorite Breadfruit Tree, I watched the plants below bend in submission from the attack of oversized raindrops.

My two sisters and my cousin stood like wooden soldiers with their backs against the tree waiting for the rain to let up. It was the beginning of the rainy season here in Cativa. There was a definite soothing magic that came along with a good rainfall that made everything still and patient in the country.

As I watched the crystal clear rain fall onto the open field, I noticed that the kids were making a mad dash towards the old country house. If only you could have been there to see the view that I had from the top of that tree. It was the closest thing to knowing what the eagle sees. It was then that I realized that the rain was not letting up, instead it had gotten heavier.

Grandma's house stood about six feet high off the ground and rested on its four wooden legs, one at each corner. Most of the houses were built high off the ground to withstand the heavy tropical rain fall that could last for days and sometimes weeks. At nights and in the dark, houses in the country are a scary sight. They looked like those slow moving mechanical robots or maybe some ancient looking space craft, as seen in some of today's motion pictures.

The rain got heavier and the leaves of my private tree gave into its force. Protection from the rain was no longer an option. I was getting soaked, so I started on my way down; carefully at first and then faster and faster. As I hurried down the wet, slippery trunk, my feet lost their grip, and I began to slide. I felt the inside of my knees, thighs and ankles meet every knot and broke every limb on the way down. I never thought that I would be so glad to feel my bottom slam against the exposed root and hard ground. My determination to get to the old house and be sheltered from the rain kept me from thinking of the pain that I was feeling.

After reaching the old country house, I inspected my body parts. All my limbs were still attached. What a surprise that was.   I was most certain that I had died and gone to heaven. With a distorted expression on her face, my sister exclaimed, "Huh! You're bleeding all over, what happened?" The two other kids steered at my bruises as if I had just contracted leprosy. With the skin now gone, the white tissue flesh was exposed. It gradually turned to a crimson color as my blood covered its surface. "What's that white stuff?", my younger sister asked. "Yuk, its turning red, look." I wiped the dirt off and cleaned my self up a bit then, we all sat on a wooden bench under the house watching the rainfall. Not much was said.

We didn't feel like much talk, but I knew that everyone would welcome a good snack. So I got a "machete" out of the tool shed and ran out to the row of pineapples. The rain felt cold to my skin as I rushed back with the head of a pineapple. I split it into four big chunks. Without peeling the skin off, we stuffed our selves until the corners of our mouths became raw and irritated.

As we continued watching the raindrops collect into puddles an idea flashed through my mind. "I know what we can do", I said to the group whose faces had gotten as gloomy as the day. "Let's play band." The announcement was like magic. It brought with it an instant dose of joy as it changed gloomy faces.

The pitter patter sound of the rain was relentless against the corrugated tin roof top as the marching band was organized. Rain water rushed into the gutter and poured down into the fifty gallon barrels located at each corner of the house. This was the reservoir of water for our family's drinking, cooking and bathing needs.

!"Miguel, you'll be the drummer O.K. All you have to do is say, bum poro bum poro bum." Miguel responded adamantly about his instrument assignment. "No, I don't wanna be the drummer. I don't wanna play the drums. I want to be the leader." I realized that Miguel was only maybe five years old, but his whining was getting to me. As stern as I could I said, "You are the smallest one here, you can't be the leader. Besides, all the other instruments are already assigned to the others." Miguel started to scream at the top of his voice. "Shah, shh." Was my immediate reaction, in an attempt to keep him quiet! "I'm gonna tell. I'm gonna tell my Ma' that you won't let me play." He continued. I wanted to strangle my cousin but, I knew that I couldn't lay a hand on him. What was worst is that he knew it too. "Alright, alright," I said in a pacifying tone. My hands were tied, anything to keep him from waking his mother. She was a pretty large woman. She seems to be always tired and required lots of rest, but when it came to discipline time you wouldn't have known it. So, I negotiated a compromise with my older sister Anita, who was assigned as band leader. "O.K. then it's set. Anita will switch parts with Miguel, Dottie you play the bugle part ta rata ta rata, got it." Turning back to Miguel, I pleaded. "And please don't you start crying again. O.K. guys lets line up. We'll march around the house once, and then we will switch parts and every body gets to play another instrument. That will make it even stevens. Miguel, you will have to play the drums later O.K." "Alright ", he replied without hesitation."Gee what a relief." I thought. He finally agreed to something without a hassle.

The band began to march in a single file formation. I was positioned at the rear of the line, beating the base drum bum, bum. Anita played the snare drums right before me, pom poro, pom poro, pom. Dottie bugled away as she marched, tata rata ,tata rata. Miguel had a hard time keeping the broom stick baton elevated above his head. The stick was taller than he was. He was constantly tripping and stumbling over it. His job as band leader was to keep us marching in step, but no one complained. He stumbled before us, and we marched out of step.

After a complete revolution of the house, the band paused to rest and trade instruments. Anita fanned her flared white cotton summer dress in an attempt to dry it out some, while Dottie pouted in a show of disgust and said, "Miguel, you are not marching right!" Within seconds an argument erupted as both girls gave Miguel instructions in the art of marching.

In the background of their argument, the subtle but most distinct symphony of percussions reached my ear. It was the music of the rain that fell on the roof top, producing thousands of hollow tin sounds. A more muffled tighter sound came from the garden as rain drops made the wide leaf plants appear to march out of step as we did. The ponds produced a quieter, but interesting tone as rain drops gave up their individualism to become pools of water. Still yet other rain drops disappeared like nails driven into a piece of wood, as they tapped and pounded themselves and finally vanished into the porous ground.

Unaware of this beguiling musical arrangement, the marching band resumed its activity. Anita was now our band leader, and Miguel had moved toward the rear of the file.

Anita was a real band leader. She had us marching in unison. She would face the band to give instructions as she marched backwards, then she would turn around lifting her knees high and thrusting the baton high above her head. Until now, things were going pretty much as expected. Little did we know that around the corner was a surprise that would change the day's events.

As she directed us around the corner of the house, her baton seemed to go into the air involuntarily. "Ooh", she cried. I rushed from the rear of the file to the corner of the house just in time to see both her legs in the air, and hear the splash she had taken into the wash tub of starching clothes. It was hilarious. She slipped while marching backwards on a slice of pineapple skin that was left on the ground and ended up in a wash-tub of starching clothes. What a funny sight, watching Anita sitting in a tub of starching clothes with her legs sticking straight up in the air.

We filled our bellies with laughter at her expense. Her feelings were hurt, and she began to sob. As I helped her out of the tub, I noticed that the dress that once was puffed out in a bell shape form now clung to her skinny legs by the weight of the sticky starch substance.

The thought of explaining this to my aunt came to mind. I hurried to help undress her, washed the starch out of the dress and hung it out to dry. We moved quickly as we gave Anita a quick bath and dressed her in some dry clothes. What we didn't realize was that it would take some time to rinse the starch out of her hair.

By the time my aunt came down stairs, I had pretty much memorized a version of what took place, but it didn't hold water. My sister, standing in a new change of clothing was explainable since it had been raining, but her hair still sticky with the starch was not, since we were forbidden to play around the work area.

"I want the truth," the stout, hefty woman remarked, towering over me in the most authoritative manner. My little bow legged cousin interrupted continually as I attempted to explain. "I should have strangled the little snitch while I had a chance", were my thoughts; since I was going to pay for it anyway. It is needless to say that I was found guilty and responsible being the oldest. My aunt executed the sentence. I did not come out smelling like a rose, but instead I got my butt starched.

The grey skies were now replaced by only blue. The chickens that had darted for shelter from the rain now paraded the grounds without a care. The plant life that once bended in submission to the pounding rain seemed to have gotten their strength back and now they stood even taller and stronger than before. My uncle got home, just in time for dinner. As he sat down he commented, "Great rain, huh kids." Only the sounds of the forks against the plates responded as we ate. The grey clouds were absorbed into the earth and now only a memory of the marching band remains.

Memoir
Perm Catheter Devil or Angel
06/12/02

A perm catheter is a connection to the vein that protrudes the body and allows a patient to receive dialysis. Since the device extends outside of the body, like an open wound, it is subject to a variety of infectious diseases. The device is intended to be temporary. Mainly installed during the maturing and healing of the main access for approximately a six months period of time.

My permanent access never matured enough to be used. A doctor explained it this way, "It was buried way too deep". It was subsequently abandoned, resulting in the continuous use of the perm catheter for two and a half years.

Because there were no needles involved in the initiation and termination of my treatment, the process was fifteen to twenty minutes faster. The connection screws on to the plastic tubing from the machine. When I saw how quickly I was put on and got out of the chair following my treatments, I thought that it wasn't a bad deal. Then I realized that I didn't have to go through the pain of getting stuck with those inch long needles every time I got dialyzed. I didn't have to wait in the chair until my blood coagulated before I could leave. It just seemed like it was an overall better deal than the needles.

For two and a half years, the only perm catheter that I ever had installed worked fine. I was to stack this experience up against the doctor's word that, I needed to get a more permanent access installed before this one gets infected.   Every one that I talked to when I traveled to different dialysis center was surprised to know that this perm catheter lasted so long. Then it finally happened. Several patients in the dialysis center, including myself, contracted some sort of staff infection. We all had perm catheter for access.

Infections to patients with perm catheters can be very dangerous because the catheter is in such a close proximity to the heart and lungs. Antibiotics are prescribed immediately to combat the infection.   Most patients recovered within the prescribed six week period that the antibiotic was given. It seemed that my infection went on for a prolonged period of forever.

I was admitted to the hospital for observation in the light of the relentless presence of this staff infection. My renal doctor did warn me that besides having to see an infection specialist, I would have to have the present perm catheter removed for fear that it may be the conduit of the infection. Well, to condense the story, I was in and out of the hospital about six times in the past two months, with the placement of three different perm catheter, which had to be replaced with as many femoral catheters.

A femoral catheter is one that is placed in the groin. It is very temporal for a single usage, maybe two. They alternated from my right to my left groin and back again to my right. One's leg must be kept immobile while the catheter is installed.   Finally, after exhausting all other possibilities for catheter installation, they went for the jugular. A inter jugular or IJ as it is referred to, is a catheter in the large vein in the neck, the jugular vain.

I recall seeing a little lady at the dialysis center some time ago now with a tube that seemed to grow from the side of her neck. She reminded me of some Borg character out of the Star Trek episodes. I never taught that I would be next on the list for assimilation.

It has been a gruesome couple of months to say the least.

The most vivid and disappointing memory that I have of this experience was with a lady surgeon. During her attempt to remove a catheter that was considered contaminated with the staff bacteria that infected my body, I received the most physical pounding and pulling on a body that I have ever seen. It just did not seem like any technique of modern medicine was employed. A friend did alert me of the physical nature of the experience that he endured with the removal of his perm catheter. Well, I could attest to it. I felt my body lift up off the table as the tiny oriental lady doctor tugged at the catheter in my chest with both hands attempting to remove it. Maybe the skin has grown over the catheter and assimilated itself into my body. If it was that doctor's body on the table, I honestly believe that a more humane procedure would be employed to extract the catheter.

One could say that a pin- cushion and I have similar characteristics, in that we have both used up with pocking. The distinction of course is that we can't accuse a pin-cushion of feeling.

Now that we have exhausted the catheter option for continued Hemo- dialysis all the doctors are pointing me in the direction of Pd, (peritoneal dialysis). Pd requires one more trip back to the hospital for yet another surgery. How silly of me to think that medicine could exist without the knife. Peritoneal dialysis is probably not the most popular of dialysis procedures.

I don't remember hearing the term Pd until I was already dialyzing, contrary to what some doctors would have you believe. They would rather remember explaining that you have a choice.

There are probably a couple of reasons why Pd is not the procedure of choice.

First of all, most emergency circumstances such as in my case, would preclude the idea of a choice. Then, we must recognize that the administration of this procedure is solely dependent on the patient. Educating the patient in the administration of this procedure is then the key factor to its success. This is not an easy proposition when there is not an economic reward to the industry. It has become the norm to convince one's self that the patient is not a good candidate for the procedure. It is much like an academician using the term uneducable, when what they really mean, is that they don't know how or that they don't want to invest the time.

I agree that quite a number of patients will opt to rely on the care given by the clinic rather than to participate in their own care and well being. But with the focus on educating the patient on how to care for them selves this number could be less.

The advantages of Pd can be significant. Patients in this program have no need to maintain regular visits to the clinic, spending four hours every day. They miss the excitement of being stuck by great big needles. They no longer have to maintain such a rigid fluid restriction. Restriction on travel lessens as well. No need to make appointments with visiting centers for dialysis, when traveling.

The disadvantages of participating in Pd are few. The most notable is the fact that the patient is now proactively engaged in his treatment. The treatment is now daily rather than every other day. The treatment is administered several times a day. Some storage of supplies is necessary. This will be my next stop. I am actually very excited about the freedom that this program will allow me. I know that I will have to be creative as to the type of work I engage myself in.

Memoir
Standing In The Sink
06/20/02

"I know you!" exclaimed the lovely young Filipino girl, as she exhibited her skill while maneuvering the push cart with the vital signs computer into the hospital room where I stayed. Her face just seemed to glow brighter as she approached and greeted me.

"Room 526", she insisted while shaking her finger at me, "You were standing in the sink". She seemed so sure of what she was saying. "No, madam it wasn't me", I defended, "I think you have got the wrong person". Her recollection of the event seemed so natural and authentic, that it had me doubting myself.

While the girl and I fenced in the middle of the room, my friend Calvin Lucky who was visiting me, rose from his chair and carefully side stepped passed us with his eyes glued to mine like metal to a magnet. He gave me a final acknowledgment with a sarcastic smirk and then said goodbye.

After my friend's departure, the nurse resumed her inquiry. "Yes, I remember you standing in the sink", she insisted. "I gave you something. Maybe tooth paste or maybe a razor."

I thought about how this young lady was a sight for sore eyes, but then she accuses me of standing in the sink. I know that I am a bit eccentric at times, but standing in the sink, no, not there yet. May I remind you reader, we are in a medical facility and not a mental health center, just in case you decided to venture off wondering.

Was she calling me crazy? Could I really have been standing in the sink while I was sedated? Am I being classified as a weirdo or a pervert? When could this have happened to me? All sorts of weird questions ran through my mind. The Filipino nurse became adamant about giving me toothpaste and watching me brush in front of the mirror and sink in my previous room 526.

So, there you have it. Her lack of command of the English language had me standing in the sink instead of at the sink. My friend Calvin Lucky had already left. How I wish that he was here to hear the explanation of this misunderstanding. Oh well, such are the entries in the annals of my life.

The following day, after returning from a perm catheter procedure that felt like fifteen men where jumping up and down and pounding on my chest for several hours, I found that I no longer held a private suit in this luxury hotel. The nurses rolled me pass a forty-two year old, Arabian man who had just been release from the intensive care unit. His name was Abraham. I know what you are thinking, but don't feel bad because I made the same mistake myself. Abraham is not Hebrew. In fact, he was quite upset when I assumed that he was.   He is a Saudi Arabian residing now in the U.S. for some time. Abraham suffered a stroke that left the left side of his body paralyzed. At first the Saudi man said very little, but by the following

187

day, we had made it pass the preliminary introduction and struggled in conversation attempting to communicate.

He explained that he was relaxing in his living room watching the evening news, when he suddenly became ill. He then tried to stand up with the intention of making his way towards the kitchen to tell his wife. The support that his legs normally provided him was no longer there.

Abraham stumbled and fell hitting every piece of furniture on the way down, before he was finally stopped by the floor. At times Abraham's speech was slurred and difficult to understand, nonetheless, his focus was not deterred. Maybe his drive comes from the fact that he holds a doctorate as a linguist, who knows what makes him tick? The fact is that he moves with a purpose, and the presence of this stroke seems to be anything more than another challenge to him.

When I first saw Abraham he was in need of a shave. His salt and pepper mustache and beard blended into the rest of the hair on his face. He had a full head of hair. His piercing black pupils seemed to smile along with the half smile of his mouth. The left side of his face showed evidence of a stroke. Part of his mouth was drawn downward in an uncontrollable fashion. He was a charming man. The nurses seemed to enjoy taking care of him; maybe it was because he ordered them around. You know how some people in a restaurant keep sending the waitress back to the kitchen for something. That is what Abraham reminds me of, but I must say that I enjoyed the direction of his conversation immensely.

Our conversations included the educational system in his country, especially the way that world geography is taught. They learned about the countries that surrounded them, followed by the rest of the countries on their continent. Their study would then proceed to the next nearest continent and so on. Another emphasis is their concentration on language. They had to learn at least, Arabic, Russian, Hebrew, and, English. Our conversation included the present Middle East conflict, and the possibility of an attack against Saadam Hussain. Thanks to his wife, we conversed without ceasing, over tea and a bowl of black seedless grapes that she graciously brought with her.

Abraham and his wife, Casey, have both had to overcome some physical challenges similar to what my wife and I have been facing. I believe that is the reason why God has brought us together, so that we might find strength and consolation in each other's experience.

Like my wife, Casey is also a breast cancer survivor. Casey described the all too familiar six weeks of radiation therapy. Abraham and I both have also been diagnosed with cancer as well. If you think that this is something, wait a minute reader. I am not finished yet. Casey will be ordained as a minister during the fall of the year, and yes you guessed it my wife, Jennie, is already a minister

189

in the service of the Lord. Casey is from Korea. In the Korean culture Casey says things occur in multiples of four, and that there are four people with similar experiences as your own.   It did not surprise her to find someone whose experiences are similar to her own.

Casey as well as anyone who has had to face the challenge of this disease knows how persistent it can be. Even when we don't see it, we cannot be too sure that it is not around. Casey knows the power of the Lord and asks that we continue to keep them in prayer.

As I mentioned earlier, Abraham is from Saudi Arabia like his mother. His father, on the other hand, is from Uzbekistan, a country in southern Russia. It is not difficult to understand the closeness that exists between Russia, Pakistan, Arabia, and the Jewish world. This is a world where adversity is common place. The will to strive and survive is embraced by its people.

Abraham's father met his mother during a business trip through the Arab world. His mother was a beautiful Arabian girl of twelve-years old, and Abraham's father was then in his thirties. She did not speak any Russian' and he did not speak any Arab. He promised her parent that he would be responsible for teaching her all the things that she needs to know, starting with the Russian language.

I taught that it seemed kind of young for his mother to marry. He reminded me that it is a different culture altogether than what I'm used to. In that part of the world, he explained, life begins early. I wished that we had more time to discuss his life further. There seems to be much of interest there.

He was released the day after I left. He had made considerable progress in recovering from that stroke. He was to continue at a physical rehabilitation center. I do have a number to reach Casey, and I promised them that I would stay in touch with them. I forgot to mention that Casey is not sitting on her duff feeling sorry for herself. She is now working on her second book. The first book will be published shortly and she is totally excited about her accomplishment. I am overjoyed for both of these individuals, as they persevere in their purpose with little regard to their circumstances.

Memoir
The Hope Of Us All
07/03/02

Last evening, I took an extended walk with my wife probably a good mile long. Although I like going for walks with her, we are so darn inconsistent that I am surprised that there is a memory. I am so blessed to have someone to share with. It was longer than previous walks. By the time we got to our destination, I was windless. She may have been kidding when she suggested that she could call our son to come and get us. I'm not so sure, but we definitely were not having that.

After getting home, we put a piece of salmon on the grill, had a nice dinner and rested.

This morning God was gracious to wake me, again, to the most beautiful sunrise against the sky. The glow of its brightness and the very warmth of its rays quickened in me a renewed reason for living. From my office window, a light breeze convinced the leaves on the aspen trees that they should dance and glisten with excitement as they bathe in the sunlight of hope.

Was it that extended walk the previous night? The grill salmon that I had! The good night sleep or was it the dawning of a new day. Whatever it was; I'm convinced that God had something to do with it. I believe that it is God's way of refreshing the spirit, rejuvenating the mind and encouraging new hope after an enduring a storm. It has been a year now since the devastating attack on the world trade center in lower Manhattan. It is true that we do not want to forget the atrocities perpetrated against us; and against our nation by evil doers, But how healthy can it be to continue to remind ourselves of the wounds and pains we have suffered. Such options keep the wounds open and make it difficult to direct our concentration towards attainable goals.

Our media seems to feed on sensationalism. Maybe I should say that we as a people have developed a veracious appetite for sensationalism. Nonetheless, we have been bombarded with headline news such as "America Fights Back", to the point of desensitization. When do we get our feelings back and abandon the apathy in our lives? Is it going to ever, be enough? Maybe we should contemplate the big picture for just a moment. It will infuse us with a reality that will bring us to the point of humbling our selves.

I recommend a very good interview of New York's Mayor, Rudy Giuliani With , Reader's Digest-The July 2002 edition, page 88, "On Guts, Glory, and What Makes America Great."

Have you ever wondered where giant leaders such as the mayor of New York City, Rudy Giuliani, get their hope and their strength? I am not a great leader like him, but, it doesn't matter how God saves your life, whether from cancer or during the tragedy of 911 you want to humble yourself before Him and serve Him. The following is Reader's Digest /Mayor Giuliani interview.

RD: Did you pray on September 11?

Giuliani: I pray at night when I go to bed-not every night, though maybe I should [laughing]. But during September 11 and after, I found myself praying in the middle of the day, asking God to help me do the right thing. I became intensely religious trying to figure things out. Why did one man live and another die? The building we were in could have been crushed by the first tower. When you contemplate those questions-the mysteries of life-it humbles you. It drives you to your knees.

RD: You have said that God spared you for a purpose.

Giuliani: God has a plan, even when you don't understand it fully. But you do have a sense of it, and you have a choice. You can conduct yourself in accordance with it or not. You can either do good or bad. I am trying to devote myself to as many good purposes as possible.

Isn't it encouraging knowing that great leaders are faced with choices similar to the ones that you and I face? What is really encouraging is that their source of strength is the same well of living water that is the hope for us all - The Christ, the Son of the living God.

In an earlier chapter I mention that I faced a dichotomy regarding my personal desire vs. God's will for my life. I also said that we would get back to that discussion later. Well, let's turn to that thought. I was saying that I knew what I wanted, but I was not too sure that God's will for my life included what I wanted.

The Bishop Acen Phillips never neglects visiting me while I have been ill. I am fortunate and blessed to have such a friend. During one of his visits to see me in the hospital, I asked for his perspective on my dilemma.

JT: Bishop, you know about my illness, and you also know about my prayers to be completely healed and restored to normal. Well I am worried that I may be praying for the wrong thing. What if it is not in His will, that I get well?

Bishop: Why would you think that it is not in God's will?

JT: I really don't know. Ever since I started coming to these clinics, I find myself encouraging other patients. It is as if I suddenly have a burden to uplift people. I also know that I want to be whole again, and my God is able.

Bishop: God always wants to hear from you. He wants you to tell him what's in your heart. He is our Father, and it gives great pleasure to see us prosper in spiritual matters first, followed by all other areas of our lives. His will is not like our will. His thoughts are not our thoughts, and His ways are not like our ways.   I don't think that there really is any contradiction between wanting to be whole again and being one who encourages others. You will have to give me a better example of what you mean.

JT: Well Bishop, what if the Lord wants me to stay and labor in this vineyard.

Bishop: And even if this was true, you don't think that you can labor in this vineyard unless you are ill. First of all, the Lord does not make any one sick. He does not want to see any one sick. He said in the Bible that He came so that you and I can have life and have it more abundantly. It sounds to me like He wants you well. The other point to consider is that the Lord wants a willing worker in the vineyard. He does not require a laborer to work against his own will. Why would He give you the gift of choice, and then be angry when you choose.

JT: Instead of praying for the recovery of my health, maybe I should be praying for the strength of my spirit to endure.

Bishop: This is good too, but you must remember that God already knows your heart. He wants you to acknowledge Him as lord of your life by coming to Him and communicating with him. He wants to give you the desires of your heart, because he loves you.

Memoir
Choosing To Return
08/12/02

Jorge Joseph Taylor

To all of you, my brothers and sisters in clinics all across the nation, dialyzing to maintain your lives, or battling against the monsters in the form of cancers, diabetes, and every other decease known to man, in effect, I write this to anyone who faces any one of life's challenges that sometimes seems to be insurmountable. Be encouraged, because God has deposited in each of you a treasure. You must look inside yourself, find it and put it to use, in spite of your circumstances.

I have been to the edge with you. Not only do I feel your pain, but I cry along with you. When the darkness came, and the night was still, and you thought that you were alone, I want you to know that I was there with you, I heard you. Yes, it is OK to have had the experience of the edge, but it is even better to be back from the edge. We must remember that we are made in the image of God. We are sons and daughters of the most - high God. We are of royal blood, but we must examine the treasure within and use it. Don't let it sit there and gather dust. Don't allow the enemy's moths to devour it.

To be able to choose is such a wonderful gift from God, directly from His image. We don't have to be sick, but we can choose to be physically or mentally challenged. As quiet as it is kept, we are all faced with some sort of challenge in this world. With some of us it is evident, with others it is not so evident, and still there are some of us that refuse to admit that we have challenges in life.

For those of us who refuse to admit or, better yet, to accept the challenges that fate has dealt us well, it really will be a hard walk, because you won't have any reason to examine your treasure. If we don't have the treasure, then it is because we don't have a personal relationship with our maker. Those of us who know Jesus as Lord, will have the treasure of His Spirit. We will be unable to contain the evidence of His love, joy, and peace, His long suffering, kindness and goodness, His faithfulness, gentleness, and self control. Only the spirit of God can deposit these gifts in our treasure chest. You can see it for yourself in the Holy Bible's New Testament, Book of Galatians, Chapter 5, verses 22-26. If you are not familiar with who Jesus is, don't be ashamed, because no one could know Him before He made it possible for us to know Him. I will again refer you to His word, which is the Holy Bible. Romans, Chapter 10 and verse 9 says this about God's righteousness, our salvation. "If you confess with your mouth the Lord Jesus, and you believe in your heart that God raised Jesus from the dead, you shall be saved." And again, my friends I invite you to check this out for yourselves. This will be your first step towards an abundant life.

I know that the walk is hard enough alone. I am concerned that you do not go it alone but I am much more concerned for the eternal circumstances of our souls. My experiences at the edge were awesome. The Lord showed me many things, among them were patience and trust. He taught me principles of warfare, such as perseverance. He thought me that the principle of fear and deceit are among the arsenal of the enemy's main weapons, and that the enemy's strong-hole is in our minds.

It is not my purpose in this book to explain all that God offers you when you become saved.

I only wanted you to see that you have a choice. Remember, that to be able to choose is Godly. God exercised His right to choose when He chose Isaac over Ishmael. Genesis 17, verse 7-8, and then again when He chose Jacob over Esau in Genesis 25, verse 9-13. Throughout the Bible there are many examples where God applies the principle of choice.

Memoir
The Peritoneal Experience
10/04/03

My Wife accused me of showing much more affection towards the new comer, Belle than to her. Of course, this was a ridiculous accusation. "How can this be", I asked myself. Whenever you see my wife you see me and vise versa, and I don't mean in a figurative sense either. I mean that we run together in the flesh.

Belle, as my wife calls it, has established itself in our lives in a most intimate way. It became surgically attached to my stomach after a medical decision that this would be my only access left to me for the purpose of dialysis.

This particular access is called peritoneal, or Pd for short, because it is placed inside the peritoneal lining of the stomach. The extended plastic tube hangs outside the stomach and this is connected nightly to a portable dialysis machine that sits next to my bed. Until the surgical implant is healed there is quite a bit of pain to the stomach area.

Much time and attention is given to the preparation of the solution, the machine, and the exit site sterilization before connecting one's, self. This process my wife refers to as, "affection towards Belle.

I remember the doctor saying that the patient must be a suitable candidate for this procedure. I actually agree with my doctor. Even though I received help from my family in various ways, for the most part, I had to be able to take care of myself in their absence. The procedure was specific. It included the following: the lifting and carrying thirty pound bags of treatment solution from their storage area to my bedside daily, engaging hand washing and catheter connectivity, utilizing aseptic techniques, understanding and maintaining the cycle dialysis machine in its proper functioning condition, maintaining a sterile environment, and changing the exit site dressing. "A suitable candidate", he said. How about including a college graduate as a suitable candidate?

Is it any wonder why this procedure may not be the most popular among the patients?

The most notable advantage in my opinion was the freedom to travel that this system allowed.

I was free to move around as long as I carried my Pd machine with me. I could take a two or three day trip taking enough fluid with me in my truck. Another option was to take a plane and have the necessary solution shipped to my destination. Once at my destination, I would set up the machine next to my bed and be ready to dialyze every night. The solution is sugar based, and I gained a few inches to my waist and of course a few pounds to my weight. Beside the freedom to travel, there was the freedom from having to visit the clinic three times a week. The psychological advantage of this freedom paid enormous dividends. I began to feel normal like most well, people who have no need of clinical visitation. It is a catch twenty two, a strange thing that the same clinic that makes you well, at the same time reminds you of how sick you are.

I suppose that there are advantages and disadvantages for different people, and people make their choice according to their circumstances. Why am I taking the peritoneal road?

You may recall the discussion earlier. We said that all dialysis patients must have what we call an access for connection to the blood line in one's body for dialysis to take place. You may also recall that the most common place for this is to be located is at an artery in the arm. In my case however, a suitable artery in this area could not be found. An onset of infection occurrences in a temporary catheter led to the choice of placing a peritoneal catheter in my stomach. In comparison to the *Hemodialysis* machine, this is considered a portable piece of equipment. It would have been nicer, had they provided a carrier with some sort of wheels. Although it is called portable, trying to get a connecting flight in a modern air port such as DIA, in Denver, or Kennedy, in New York, or the Mid Way in Chicago is challenging enough for the "normal" individual with the single allowable carry on baggage. I had to carry my luggage in addition to the dialysis machine.

The drawback of this peritoneal catheter probably as well as any type of catheter is its susceptibility to infections.

The experience with the Peritoneal Dialysis was kind of different. It was kind of the adult version of dialysis. What I mean by that is that no one is there to watch you. You either did the procedures right or suffered the consequences. It was as simple as that. The reward for being a model student was like being handed back the reign of your destiny, along with a relative amount of freedom.

I believe that I appeared the healthiest on this system. I certainly felt better after each treatment. Not having to go to the clinic every other day was a prize in itself. Those of you who must make that every other day commute to the clinic know exactly what I mean. I have mentioned this before. As much as we are grateful and understand the life giving service provided by the clinic, its appearance tends to remind me more of the Old Testament leper colonies. The self confidence that comes, because of the personal involvement of one's own care, was priceless.

We are all aware that a coin has two sides that we have labeled heads and tails. The heads side of the coin is more favorable, but it is accompanied by the tail, and so it is with the peritoneal dialysis. You must be prepared with a storage location in your house to accommodate a month's supply of solution. There are two fifteen-pound bags of solution per box. One box is usually a daily prescription. If you live in an apartment, space might be a premium, and this may not be an option for you. Now, if you happened to be living in a house, but your bedroom is not conveniently located on the main floor, then you have got to figure out a way of getting a thirty-pound box

Jorge Joseph Taylor

of solution to your bedroom every day. Having managed to get a week's supply of fluid upstairs, you begin to see the transformation of your bedroom and house with the appearance of boxes everywhere. It seems like you are always packing, getting ready to move. To add to the clutter even more, you connect a twenty-five foot plastic tube from your bedside to your bathroom. If you are not in the master bedroom, then your plastic tube is going across the main hall way to hang inside the toilet bowl of your main bathroom.

Sleeping with the tubes attached to my stomach was not much fun. First off, it was very uncomfortable no matter what was done to alleviate it. The machine sat on my nightstand to the left of my bed, and that forced me to sleep on the left side of my body. Sleeping on my back was terrible. All the fluid in my stomach seems to crush my lungs making me unable to breath. This just did not seem like any humane choice for existence. At times, I felt like a mouse of a person because certainly there must be people who are making it under this condition without complaining.   The machine's alarm is relentless through the night. Forget a full night's rest. No such thing. The concern here was how do I keep my neighbors from calling the cops on me, because I am not in compliance with the neighborhoods noise ordinance? Just kidding, the fact is that I have very nice neighbors.

If you are blessed with a mate and have managed to sell her or him on this peritoneal system being the best thing for your household, notice that I said household and not just you, after all that I have mentioned thus far, you are most definitely blessed.

It is most definitely a personal choice whether or not one chooses peritoneal over hemodialysis. It is my intention to present as much information or facts so that making choices would be done as intelligently as possible.

I left the worst for last. I want to inform you now about the infections that are the enemy of the Pd catheter. Maybe I should say that infections are not exclusive enemies to pd it only seems that way when this is your access choice. Once an infection gets into the peritoneum more often than not, the catheter has to be removed to be sure that the infection is completely removed. No amount of sedative seems to alleviate the pain in one's stomach. If I understood my doctor correctly, he mentioned that there were three different types of infections: bacterial, viral and infections that are a fungus. Of these three the fungus infection is the one that is feared the most. The reason that it is feared the most is that the fungus is alive and grows and hides to avoid extinction from antibodies. It learns to become immune to antibodies. In general, it can be a challenge that can be lost in many cases. I managed to contract a fungus infection that landed me in the hospital.

The catheter in my peritoneum had to be removed to insure that the infection would be totally eliminated.

The fungus infection caused some bleeding of the fluids from my peritoneum into my blood stream. Because the dialyzing fluid is sugar based, it resulted in an elevated sugar level beyond six hundred. I was placed immediately on a diabetic diet and medication. Three times a day, after testing my blood sugar content, I had to give myself insulin shots to help bring those numbers down. After about a month of treatment, my sugar level was brought within a controllable 150 and stayed there.

This mode of dialysis was very interesting. One has to be truly committed to care for one's self. There is no nurse or technicians to put you on the machine or take you off. There is no professional to see that you get your medication during every run as with hemodialysis. There is a visit to the clinic a couple of times a month to assess the effectiveness of the dialysis, and to get examined by the doctor.

Maybe Pd is not for me right at this moment. Don't get me wrong, I love the freedom that comes along with it. It's just that right, now I'm not as dedicated to my care as I need to be.

Dialyzing at home is now a thing of the past at least for the present. I have returned to my Monday, Wednesday and Friday clinical dialysis schedule.

Memoir
Ron Is Gone
12/05/03

"Ron's gone", were the words from one of the technicians that greeted me one Wednesday afternoon as I approached the scale to weigh myself as we are required to do before beginning our dialysis run. Most people would know the meaning behind those words. "What do you mean by Ron's gone", was my response, as if there could be some other meaning to those words.

It was said that Ron had a good run on the Friday before everything seem to go just right, then came the weekend, and on Monday Ron didn't return to dialysis. Sometime over the weekend, his heart had stopped. He died of a heart attack.

He was so young. He was only thirty-five years old, and seemed to be full of promise. He had a transplant that didn't work for some reason, but Ron was really excited and full of hope for this new transplant. As long as there is time, we who are left in it, must keep on marching, until we are free from time.

There is not one thing that Ron can do about being gone. It is too late.

Since Ron's death, I have often times thought about him and asked questions such as: "Was he satisfied with the accomplishments of his life? Did he affect the people that he intended to share with? Did he realize the purpose of his life? Did he come to know Christ? At times he really did not appear to be ill. What does it all mean? It doesn't seem to matter whether you are ill or whether health is on your side. Pastor Del Phillips explained it this way during one of his sermons, "The fact is that we are all on the same course with the same end in time. The same course means that our faith and our end in time are predetermined. Maintaining the same course means that the discovery of events and landmarks along the way, will all be common and unavoidable. We will all experience the same events, and the end of the trail will be the same for all of us, unless we change our course of travel."

I don't know the answers to these questions! The reason that I don't know is because I did not take the time to become involved. Maybe this indicts me. I must do better next time. I am sure that I will have the opportunity to share with someone else if I maintain this course in time. I was humanly affected by crossing Ron's path.

Memoir
Championing The Cause
09/25/02

Jorge Joseph Taylor

A couple of days ago I walked into the dialysis center for treatment, and I was greeted by a poster picture of Danny Glover in the waiting room of the center. Mr. Glover has been selected as a spokesperson for ESRD, better known as kidney failure disease by the National Kidney Foundation. I was delighted to see that finally a spokesperson had been selected to champion such a cause.

It just seems like activity towards promoting public awareness and education about the effects of this disease has been slow coming. I often wonder if it is because African Americans and people of color have been the most affected victims of ESRD, similarly to diabetes, hypertension, and Sickle cell anemia.

ESRD is a disease that can be very misleading or misunderstood. Victims of this disease can sometimes appear healthy and normal. I have had individuals tell me that I do not look sick, or how well I look considering my ailment. I have also heard people refer to individuals who are unable to continue with their conventional jobs, because of their kidney illness, as slackers. This perspective about the disease is held by the public as well as by some patients with the disease.

The range of appearances can be as different as day is from night. Some patient's quality of life changes very little, while others with the same disease can find themselves in a much more diminished life style. I have seen patients hop onto a motor cycle and speed away from the center at the end of their treatment; while others are helped with their prosthetics and into their wheel chairs.

My message in writing this book is two fold. First, to the challenged individual, whether it be by kidney failure, heart, lungs, diabetes, MS or any other circumstance that limits your world, we must not forget that coping is essential to our survival. We must find the source that allows us to keep going. I have shared my own experiences in the hope that God allowed a revelation that may be helpful in your challenging walk.

My second reason is to appeal to the families, friends and neighbors who up until now have never thought of being champions of a cause. I hope that I have made you curious enough about kidney failure to seriously consider what you can do to help make it easier for those who must face these challenges.

If you are asking yourself, where do you start? , or what can you do?, well being an organ donor is the simplest way that I know. Especially since at the present time, there is a waiting list for kidney transplants about four years out. All you need to do is tell the clerk at the time of renewing your driver's license that you want to be a donor. You may also become a living anonymous donor. I urge you to inquire with the folks down at the National Kidney Foundation about other ways to assist, and be a champion of this cause.